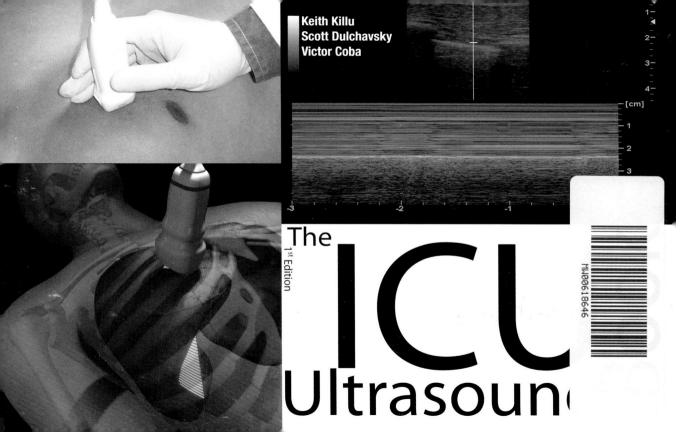

Keith Killu
Scott Dulchavsky
Victor Coba

The
1ST Edition
ICU
Ultrasoun

MW00618646

Art/Design/Photography, Surgical Imagineers at Butler Graphics, Inc.
3D Modeling, Butler Graphics/VitalPxl Collaboration
Male/Female 3D Model, Zygote

Dedication

I dedicate this small measure of work to
   My Mother, for all your sacrifices
   My Wife, for always being there
   And
   All Ultrasound enthusiasts on earth and in space.
                  Keith Killu MD, Detroit

Dedicated to my wife, who first showed me the value of ultrasound,
and to the frontier astronaut and cosmonaut sonographers on the International Space Station who inspired us to expand the indications
and education for point of care ultrasound.
                  Scott A. Dulchavsky MD PhD, Detroit

To my sweetheart and family for their love, support and patience throughout the entire project and the inspiration for upcoming future
endeavors.
                  Victor Coba MD, Detroit

Leads

Keith Killu MD, FCCP, FACP
Clinical Assistant Professor/
Wayne State University School of
Medicine

Critical Care medicine/Dept. of
Surgery, Henry Ford Hospital

Scott A. Dulchavsky MD,PhD
Professor/Wayne State University
School of Medicine

Chairman/Dept. of Surgery, Henry
Ford Hospital

Victor Coba MD
Critical Care Medicine/Emergency
Medicine
Staff Physician/Dept. of Emergency
Medicine
Henry Ford Hospital

Authors

Karthikeyan Ananthasubramaniam MD, FACC,FASE
Associate Professor of Medicine/
Wayne State University School of
Medicine
Director of Nuclear Cardiology and
Echo cardiography Lab/
Dept. of cardiology, Henry Ford Hospital

David Amponsah MD
Assistant Clinical Professor/Wayne State
University School of Medicine
Ultrasound Director/
Dept. of Emergency Medicine,
Henry Ford Hospital

J. Antonio Bouffard MD
Senior Staff Radiologist/
Bone Radiology Division
Department of Diagnostic Radiology,
Henry Ford Hospital

Brian M. Craig MD
Ultrasound Section Leader
Dept. of Radiology,
Henry Ford Hospital

Kathleen Garcia FASE, RVT
Wyle Integrated Science & Engineering
Houston, Texas

Patrick R. Meyers BS, RDMS,RDCS, RVT
Owner
Musculoskeletal Ultrasound of Wisconsin

Jennifer Milosavljevic MD
Staff Physician
Dept. of OB/GYN,
Henry Ford Hospital

Luca Neri, MD
Professor/USCME Project Director
Past President, WINFOCUS
Critical Care
A. O. Niguarda Ca' Granda Hospital
Milano, Italy

Kathleen O'Connell
Medical Student
Wayne State University School of
Medicine
Detroit, Michigan

Ashot Sargsyan, MD
Wyle Integrated Science & Engineering
Houston, Texas

Enrico Storti, MD
USCME Project Codirector, WINFOCUS
Critical Care
A. O. Niguarda Ca' Granda Hospital
Milano, Italy

Guillermo Uriarte RN,RDCS,RCVT
Technical Director, Lead Echo
Sonographer
Dept. of Noninvasive Cardiology
Henry Ford Hospital

Gabiele Via, MD
Editorial Board/Critical Ultrasound Journal
Department of Anesthesia & Intensive
Care
University of Pavia • Pavia, Italy

Contributors

Jack Butler
Media Specialist, Surgical Imagineer
Dept. of Surgery/Henry Ford Hospital
Butler Graphics, Inc., CEO

Neil Rudzinski
Media Specialist 3D Visualization
Dept. of Surgery/Henry Ford Hospital

Volunteers

Peter Altshuler
Alexandria Dulchavsky
Caitlin Reddy
Michael Nowak

Table of Contents

Abbreviations

AO	Aorta
AV	Aortic Valve
CCA	Common Carotid Artery
CBD	Common Bile Duct
CCW	Counterclockwise
CF	Color Flow
CFA	Common Femoral Artery
CFV	Common Femoral Vein
CHD	Common Hepatic Duct
CW	Clockwise
DCM	Dilated Cardiomyopathy
DFV	Deep Femoral Vein
ET	Endotracheal
FV	Femoral Vein
GB	Gallbladder
GSV	Greater Saphenous Vein
HOMC	Hypertrophic Obstructive Cardiomyopathy
IJV	Internal Jugular Vein
Inn	Innominate
IVC	Inferior Vena Cava
IVS	Interventricular Septum
LA	Left Atrium
LLQ	Left Lower Quadrant
LUQ	Left Upper Quadrant
LV	Left Ventricle
LVOT	Left Ventricuar Outflow Tract
MV	Mitral Valve
ON	Optic Nerve
ONSD	Optic Nerve Sheath Diameter
PAP	Pulmonary Artery Pressure
PE	Pulmonary Embolus
PEA	Pulseless Electrical Activity
PFA	Profunda Femoris Artery
PI	Pulmonary Incompetence
PR	Pulmonary Regurgitation
PV	Pulmonary Valve
PW	Pulsed Wave Doppler
RA	Right Atrium
RAP	Right Atrial pressure
RLQ	Right Lower Quadrant
RUQ	Right Upper Quadrant
RV	Right Ventricle
RVIT	Right Ventricular Inflow Tract
RVOT	Right Ventricular Outflow Tract
SCV	Subclavian Vein
SFA	Superficial Femoral Artery
SFV	Superficial Femoral Vein
SVC	Superior Vena Cava
TV	Tricuspid Valve
US	Ultrasound

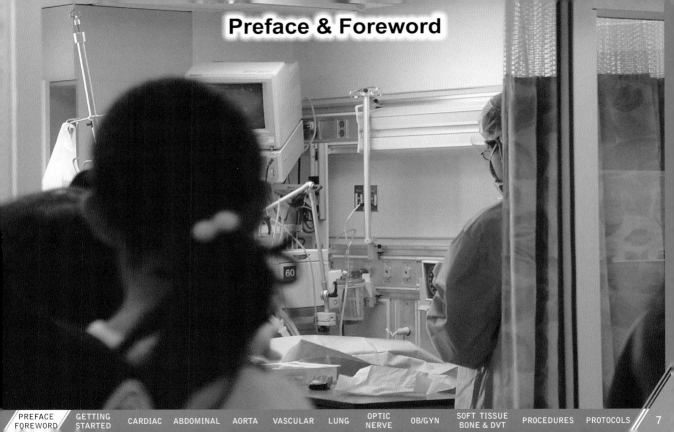

Preface

The ICU Ultrasound pocket book is far and above the most concise, targeted reference source to enable the novice or advanced emergency or ICU clinician to incorporate point of care ultrasound into their practice. This book effectively teams internationally recognized sonologists with NASA researchers developing just in time ultrasound training methods for astronauts on the International Space Station, to provide a rapid ultrasound diagnostic and procedural guide for the ICU. The comprehensive sections included in this book cover the ever expanding array of clinical indications for non-radiologist performed ultrasound and provide a novel addition to this field.

Scott A. Dulchavsky MD PhD

Detroit 2010

Foreword

Bedside intensivist-performed ultrasonography easily qualifies as one of the most, if not the most important paradigm shifting technology developed in critical care in recent years. The availability of less expensive, smaller machines with better resolution has made bedside examination by the intensivist feasible. What is it about bedside ultrasonography that is so compelling for the ICU physician? Ultrasonography permits the "ultimate" physical examination. It allows immediate assessment of vital cardiopulmonary, abdominal, renal, and vascular structural and functional elements in the unstable patient. Considerably less diagnostic guess work results in a more precise workup, with less unnecessary, and potentially hazardous, transports to radiology. Furthermore it replaces "blind" or landmark guided procedures with defined anatomic visualization that translates into safer, faster, and less painful procedures.

Critical Care physicians have been slower than their Emergency Medicine colleagues to adopt this technology, but this is changing rapidly. There is an expanding literature on the use of ultrasonography in critically ill patients. Recent consensus guidelines outlining specific elements of knowledge that define competency in critical care ultrasound have been published. Training guidelines and examinations designed to demonstrate proficiency in critical care ultrasonography are the next steps to fully establishing intensivist-performed ultrasound.

This book succeeds outstandingly in one important part of that process: the creation of educational materials designed to be used at the ICU bedside to guide image acquisition, image interpretation, and procedural ultrasound. As such "The ICU Ultrasound Pocket Book" is a valuable resource for medical students, nurses, physician extenders, residents, and fellows, as well as practicing intensivists.

> John M. Oropello, MD, FCCM, FCCP, FACP
> Program Director, Critical Care Medicine
> Professor of Surgery & Medicine
> Mount Sinai School of Medicine
> New York, N.Y.

Getting Started
Equipment, Knobology & Terminology

Ashot Sargsyan, MD
Kathleen Garcia, FASE, RVT

Advantages of Ultrasound
- Noninvasive
- Highly feasible
- Rapid, versatile & repeatable
- Time saving

Be familiar with your ultrasound machine

Knobology may be presented differently by different machines, but the principle is the same

Setting the machine initially to obtain the best sonographic picture is of ultimate importance

The learning curve is usually steep

Contents

Transducers

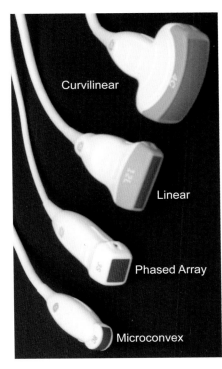

The transducer contains a piezoelectric material or crystal that has the ability to convert electricity to US waves as well as converting the returning waves into electric signals.

The new transducers are array transducers that contain crystals or groups of crystals arranged along the footprint.

Sequential array transducers refer to sequential activation of each crystal. The linear and curvilinear tranducers are usually of this type.

Phased array tranducers use a group of crystals and using every element with each US pulse. The cardiac transducer is an example of this type.

Curvilinear Transducer
Frequency ranges 2-5 MHz
Larger, curved footprint with excellent penetration for deeper structures and great lateral resolution

Usually used for abdominal exam

Linear Transducer
Frequency ranges 7-13 MHz
High resolution for superficial structures. Poor penetration for deep structures
Used for vascular, lung, musculoskeletal, nerves and optic exams

Phased Array (Cardiac) Transducer
Frequency ranges 2.5-5 MHz
Smaller flat footprint with medium resolution for superficial structures and a better penetration for deeper structures

Used for cardiac, lung and abdominal exams

Microconvex Transducer
Frequency ranges about 4-11 MHz
Smaller footprint with medium resolution for superficial structures and a better penetration for deeper structures
General use in adult patients is for abdominal, lung and vascular exams

Basic US Machine Layout

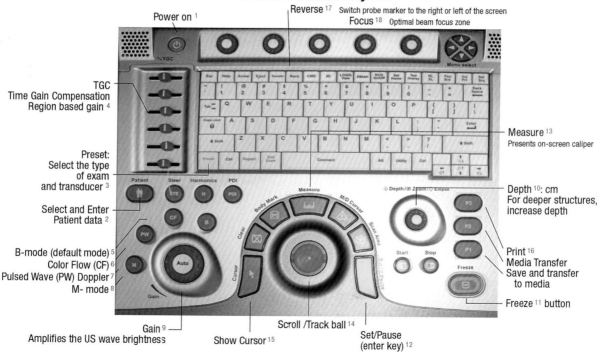

Power on [1]

Reverse [17] Switch probe marker to the right or left of the screen

Focus [18] Optimal beam focus zone

TGC
Time Gain Compensation
Region based gain [4]

Preset:
Select the type
of exam
and transducer [3]

Select and Enter
Patient data [2]

B-mode (default mode) [5]
Color Flow (CF) [6]
Pulsed Wave (PW) Doppler [7]
M- mode [8]

Measure [13]
Presents on-screen caliper

Depth [10]: cm
For deeper structures,
increase depth

Print [16]
Media Transfer
Save and transfer
to media

Freeze [11] button

Gain [9]
Amplifies the US wave brightness

Show Cursor [15]

Scroll /Track ball [14]

Set/Pause
(enter key) [12]

	US Machine/Controls	
1.	**Power**	Turn Power on and off
2.	**Patient**	Select, enter and edit Patient data
3.	**Preset**	To select a preprogrammed setting for a given type of exam and transducer
4.	**TGC**	Time Gain Compensation. Adjusts the gain at different depths
5.	**B-mode (default mode)**	Brightness mode. Live gray scale image of all structures. Also known as 2D modes
6.	**Color Flow (CF)**	Also known as Color Doppler mode. Detects fluid flow and direction
7.	**Pulsed Wave (PW) Doppler**	Displays live blood flow spectrum vs. time at the PW Cursor site (in the heart or a vessel), to reveal flow direction, laminarity, velocities and indices
8.	**M-mode**	The motion mode. Displays motion of anatomical structures in time along the M-mode cursor.
9.	**Gain**	Amplifies the US wave brightness
10.	**Depth**	Adjust the depth to focus on the organ being examined . For deeper structures, increase the depth
11.	**Freeze**	Display shows image snapshot
12.	**Set/Pause**	Acts similar to a computer mouse button
13.	**Measurement**	Initiates measurement by bringing up calipers (mode- and preset-specific)
14.	**Scroll**	Track ball
15.	**Cursor**	Press to make the cursor appear and disappear
16.	**Print & Media Transfer button**	Save and transfer data to media keys
17.	**Reverse**	Switch screen indicator to the right and left of the screen
18.	**Focus**	Focuses the US beam at the depth of interest for better resolution and image quality

Definitions	
Wave length:	The distance an US wave travels in one cycle
Frequency:	The number of times a wave is repeated per second. 1 Hz= 1 wave cycle/sec. Common diagnostic US frequency is 2-12 million (mega) Hz ,(MHz)
Acoustic power:	The amount of energy emitted by the transducer
ALARA:	As Low As Reasonably Achievable. This principle must be followed to minimize the probability of bio-effects of acoustical energy on tissues
Grayscale:	The principle of assigning levels of gray (usually 256 levels from white to black) to the returning US pulses according to their intensity. Strongly reflecting anatomical structures are more echogenic, while non-reflecting areas are non-echogenic.
Reflection:	Redirection of portion of the US wave to its source
Refraction:	Redirection of the US wave as it crosses a boundary between two mediums with different densities (acoustical properties)
Spatial Resolution	Ability of the machine to image finer detail. Measured by the ability to identify closely spaced structures as separate entities.
Axial Resolution:	The ability to differentiate between two closely spaced structures that lie parallel to the US beam. Can be improved by using a higher frequency transducer
Lateral resolution:	The ability to differentiate between two closely spaced structures at the same depth. Can be improved with adjusting the focal zone

Modes

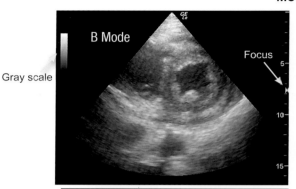

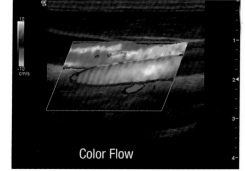

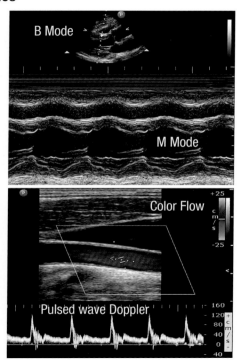

Modes

Color Flow orientation

When applying Color Flow, the top of the box on the left or right of the screen will indicate the color of the flow towards the transducer, and the bottom of the box indicates the color of the flow away from the transducer. In this example the flow towards the transducer is red, and the flow away from the transducer is blue.

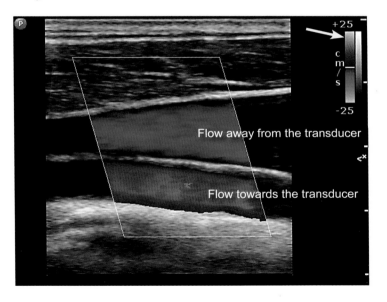

Controls
Gain

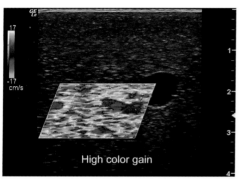

High color gain

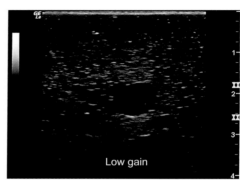

Low gain

Depth

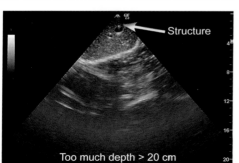

Structure

Too much depth > 20 cm

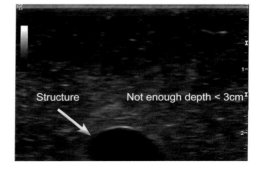

Structure

Not enough depth < 3cm

Image Orientation

Structures should be examined in two orthogonal planes, commonly transverse (axial, horizontal) and longitudinal (either sagittal or coronal).

If a transverse image (cross section) is being obtained, place the transducer marker towards the patient's right, and make sure the US monitor indicator is in default position (to the left of the screen)

- Structures located near the transducer marker will appear near the marker on the screen
- This US image project structures on the right side of the patient to the left side of the screen, similar to a CT image

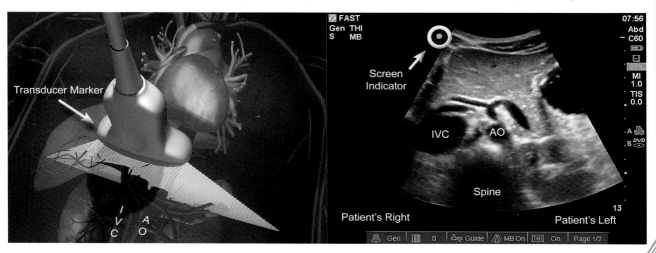

Image Orientation

If a longitudinal image (sagittal) is being obtained, place the transducer marker towards the patient's head (cephalad) and make sure the US monitor indicator is in default position (to the left of the screen)

This will project structures closest to the patient's head on the left side of the screen.

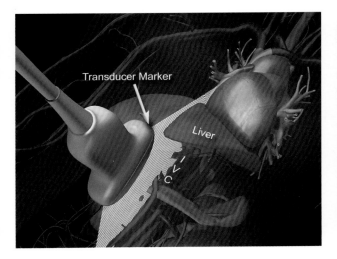

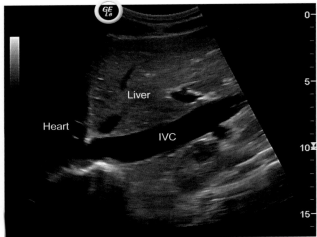

Terminology

Echoic

A relative characteristic of an US image area that contains echos .

The Liver image is often used as a reference to describe adjacent image areas as "hypoechoic" or "hyperechoic"

Anechoic/Black

Image areas with no echos (black)

Usually representing structures filled with uniform fluid.

"Acoustical shadows" from a bone or calculus may also be anechoic

Hypoechoic/Light Grey

Darker gray areas, as compared to the liver image as reference

Isoechoic/Grey

The level of gray equals to the reference area or the surrounding tissue.

Often compared to the liver image as a reference

Hyperechoic/White

Lighter gray areas as compared to the reference area or the surrounding tissue

Often compared to the liver image as a reference

Examples are fascial layers, calcified areas and bone surfaces, reverberation from gas-containing structures and some image artifacts

Artifact

Spurious patterns on the US image (often hyperechoic) that do not correspond topographically to anatomical structures

Usually extends to the top of the screen

Interrupted by air and bony structures

Moves with the movement of the transducer

Acoustic shadow

Anechoic or hypoechoic shadow in the projected path of the US beam after it encounters a highly reflective surface (e.g. calculus or bone)

Mirror Image

A duplicate image of the structure appearing on both sides of a strong reflector (e.g., diaphragm)

Reverberation Artifact

An abnormal recurrent hyperechoic pattern of equal distances

Occurs when the US wave is "trapped" and bounces between two reflective interfaces

Terminology

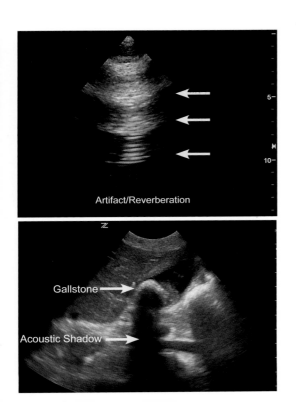

Artifact/Reverberation

Gallstone

Acoustic Shadow

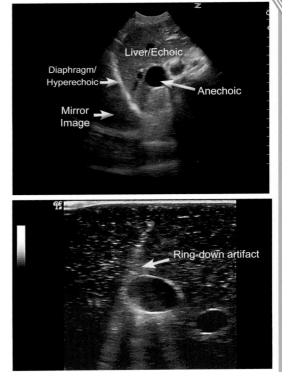

Liver/Echoic

Diaphragm/Hyperechoic

Anechoic

Mirror Image

Ring-down artifact

Transducer Orientation

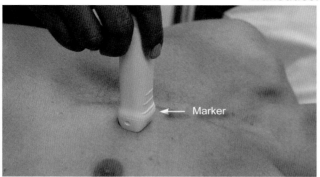

Marker

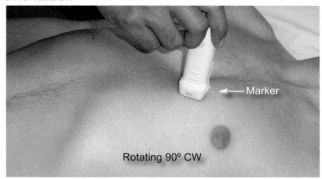

Marker

Rotating 90° CW

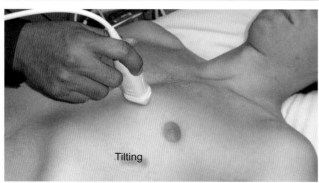

Tilting

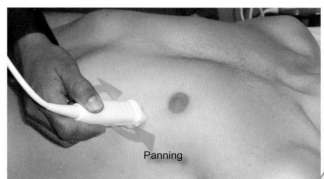

Panning

Getting Started

Operating the US machine has the same basic principles with all manufacturers. Familiarize yourself with your machine

Formulate a question to be answered by the US examination, for example:

- Is there pleural effusion?
- What is the LVED volume status?
- Is there an increase in the ICP?
- What is the safest path for a vein access?

Prepare the US machine, the transducer needed, gel and sterile sheath if needed before starting the exam

Place the US machine by the bedside with the screen in comfortable visual contact

Avoid excessive lighting

Getting Started
1. Turn on the machine
2. Enter Patient data
3. Select a transducer (Preset Button)
4. Start with all TGC sliders in the midline as a standard and change as needed
5. Start in B Mode. All machines have the B Mode (2D) as default
6. Place the screen indicator to the left of the screen (default), except in cardiac exam it should be on the right. The indicator position will change when using the Reverse button Apply enough gel on the transducer
7. Start US exam
8. Adjust the Gain
9. Adjust the Depth so that the structure examined fits the view and fills the center of the screen. Note the depth on the right of the screen
10. Use the focus to improve the image quality of the desired structure
11. Continue US scanning and have fun

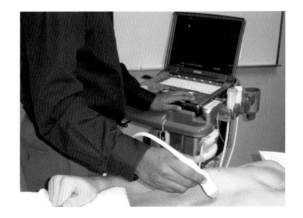

Cardiac Exam

Keith Killu, M.D.
Karthikeyan Ananthasubramaniam, MD
Guillermo Uriarte, RN

Contents

Primary indications

Evaluation of global cardiac function
Estimation of intravascular volume status
Detection of Pericardial Effusion and Cardiac Tamponade
LV & RV systolic function evaluation
Evaluation of wall motion
Evaluation of valve function

Extended Indications

Evaluation of CVP
Evaluation of IVC
Evaluation of PAP
Evaluation of the proximal aorta for dissection/aneurysm

Terminology

2D image (B mode): Brightness mode for anatomical assessment

M mode: motion assessment of a structure over time. Distance & depth measurements are usually done with this mode

Color flow Doppler (CF): For hemodynamic and anatomical information

Continuous Wave (CW) and Pulsed Wave (PW) Doppler: For hemodynamic assessment, calculating velocity and pressure gradients

Cine loop: frame to frame assessment

Cardiac Package: Usually included with the software for calculations

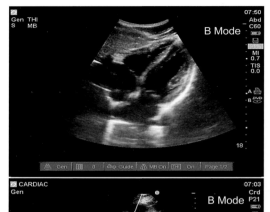

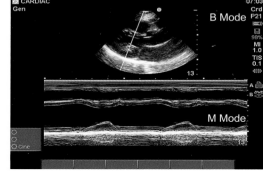

Patient position/Control Settings/ Transducers

Patient Position   Most critically ill patient have to be examined in a supine position. If possible a left lateral position will improve the cardiac window in the parasternal and apical views by pushing the heart closer to the chest wall

Control Settings   The **Screen indicator** is placed to the **"Right"** of the screen

The depth should be set at about **15 cm** then adjust as needed

Start with the B Mode

Transducer Type   Phased Array (Cardiac) transducer

2.5-5 MHz

Small and can fit between the ribs

Curvilinear (abdominal) transducer

2-5 MHz

Mostly for subcostal view during the FAST exam

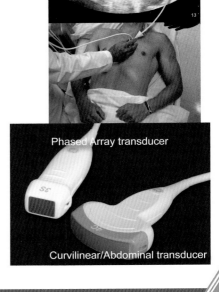

Phased Array transducer

Curvilinear/Abdominal transducer

Echocardiographic Windows

Transducer Positions/ C = Cardiac

The following windows should be considered only as a guide for transducer position and marker orientation. They can vary from patient to patient and by patient position

C1= Parasternal Window

- About the 3rd or 4th intercostal space, left sternal border
- Footprint pointing towards the spine
- Long axis= Transducer marker at 10 o'clock
- Short axis= Transducer marker at 2 o'clock

C2= Apical Window

- About the 5th or 6th intercostal at the point of maximal impulse
- Footprint pointing towards the right shoulder
- 4 chamber= Transducer marker at 3 o'clock
- 5 chamber = Transducer marker at 3 o'clock with slight tilting of the footprint upward
- 2 chamber= Transducer marker at about 12 o'clock

C3= Subcostal Window

- Below the Xiphoid process
- Footprint towards the left shoulder

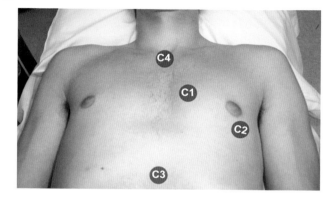

- 4 chamber= Transducer marker at 3 o'clock
- Short axis= Transducer marker at 6 o'clock
- IVC= Footprint towards the spine and the transducer marker at 6 o'clock, in cardiac presets or 12 o'clock in abdominal/general presets

C4= Suprasternal Window

- At the Suprasternal notch
- Footprint towards the back of the sternum (Inferior & Posterior)
- Long axis= Transducer marker at 2 o'clock
- Short axis= Transducer marker at 3 - 5 o'clock

Parasternal Window/Long Axis View

Left Parasternal Long Axis View

This is usually the first window and somewhat easier to obtain

Transducer Position

C1

Transducer marker pointing towards the patient's right shoulder

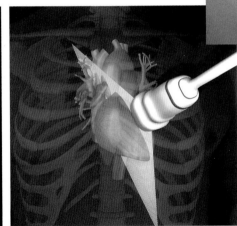

Marker

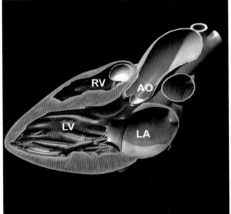

Parasternal Window/Long axis
Myocardial segments

Sonographic Findings

Note the overall activity of the heart and any gross abnormality

Note any pericardial effusion especially below the posterior wall

Examine the cardiac segments motion and structure

1. Posterior basal and middle
2. Apical inferior and anterior
3. Septal
4. RV Wall

Myocardial segments may be dysfunctional during acute myocardial infarction

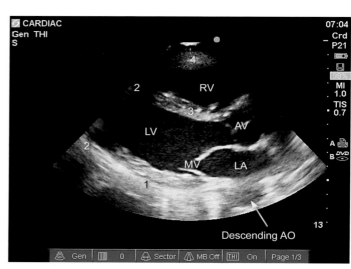

Descending AO

Parasternal Window/Long axis
Valvular function

Sonographic Findings (cont.)

Use Color Flow **(CF)** to identify and evaluate the mitral and aortic valve function and detect any abnormality

Note any valvular dysfunction, note any significant stenosis or regurgitation

Blood moving in multiple directions will display **variance** and different multiple colors

Note any papillary muscle or chordae tendineae rupture

Large valve vegetations can be seen

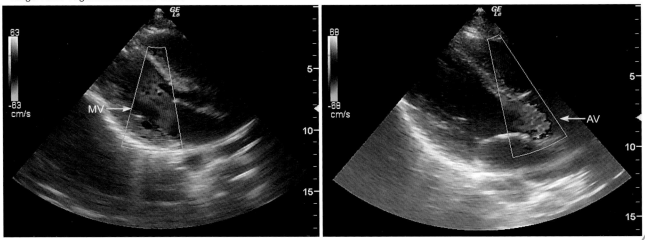

Parasternal Window/Long axis
Valvular function

Aortic Valve

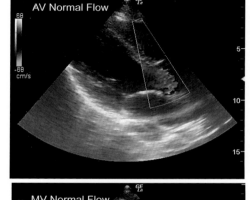

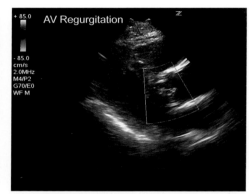

Mitral Valve

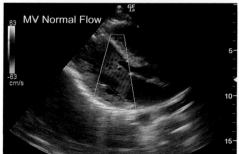

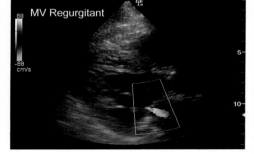

Parasternal Window/Short axis View

Transducer Placement

Start location: **C1**

From the long axis view turn the marker towards left shoulder [i.e. turn 90° CW]

Start with the transducer footprint perpendicular to the skin to obtain the round shaped **"Donut"** image of the Short axis

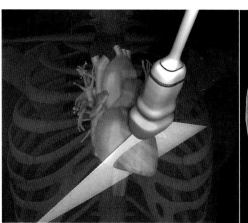

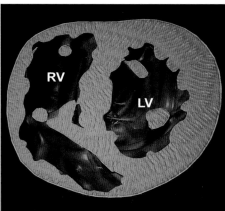

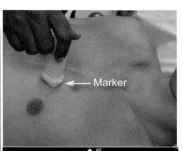

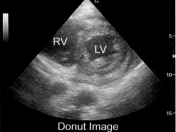

Donut Image

Parasternal Window/Short axis View – Apex

Transducer Placement

Start location: **C1**

Transducer tilted downward with the footprint pointing towards the left thigh to obtain a short axis image at the apical level

Sonographic Findings

To evaluate the myocardial segments and note any **apical hypokinesis**

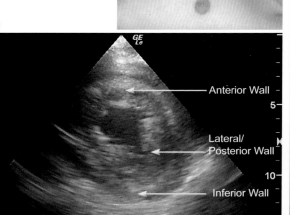

Marker

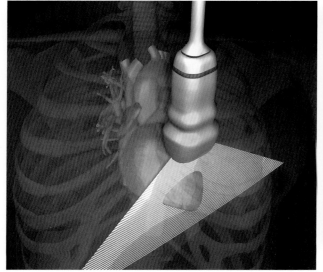

Anterior Wall

Lateral/ Posterior Wall

Inferior Wall

Apical Segment

Parasternal Window/Short axis View – Papillary M

Transducer Placement

Start location: **C1**

From the apical position, tilt the transducer upward moving towards the right shoulder to obtain a Papillary muscle view **"Donut"**. The footprint will be almost perpendicular to the skin

Sonographic Findings

This view is used to assess the fluid status and **EF by the "eyeballing"** method

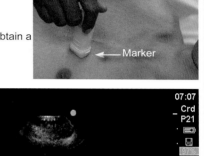

← Marker

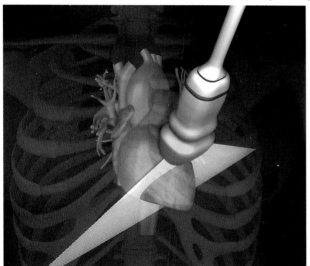

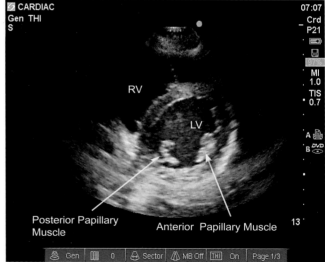

CARDIAC
Gen THI
S
07:07
Crd
P21
MI 1.0
TIS 0.7

RV

LV

Posterior Papillary Muscle

Anterior Papillary Muscle

13

Gen | 0 | Sector | MB Off | THI On | Page 1/3

Parasternal Window/Short axis
Papillary M/Myocardial segments

Sonographic Findings (cont.)

Examine the myocardial segments and wall motion

1. Anterior
2. Septal
3. Inferior
4. Posterior/Lateral

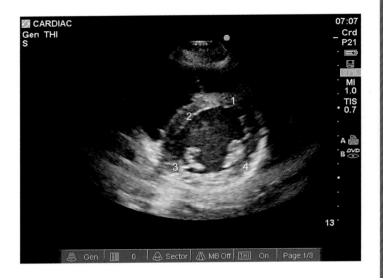

Parasternal Window/Short axis View – Mitral Valve

Transducer Placement

Start location: **C1**

From the position of the papillary muscles, by tilting the transducer upward towards the right shoulder, a view of the mitral valve can be obtained

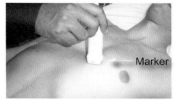
Marker

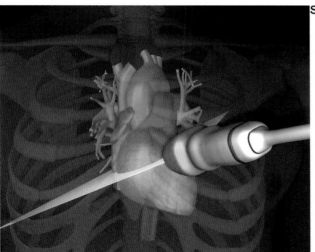

Sonographic Findings

* Note the **"Fish Mouth"**
* Examine MV function
* Note any severe stenosis
* Examine the wall segments

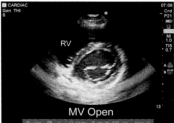
RV
MV Open

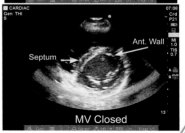
Septum
Ant. Wall
MV Closed

Parasternal Window/Short axis View – AV & RVOT

Transducer Placement

Start location: **C1**

From the position of the MV, angling the transducer upward with the footprint towards the right shoulder, a view of the **Aortic valve** and the **RVOT** can be obtained

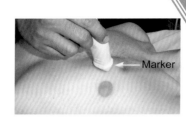

Marker

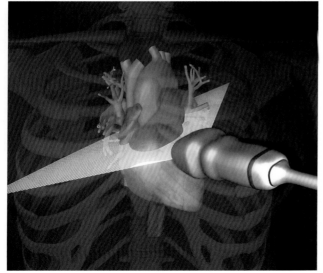

Sonographic Findings

- Examine AV and PV function and note any severe stenosis
- Note the **Mercedes-Benz** sign representing the AV

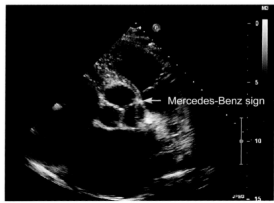

Mercedes-Benz sign

Parasternal Window/Short axis
AV & RVOT

Sonographic Findings (cont.)

Examine the AV, RVOT and the PV

Use CF to examine for any **PI**, which can help in the measurement of the Pulmonary artery pressure **(PAP)** by Doppler method

Examine the main PA for regurgitation

Examine the right and left PA

May be able to detect a large **pulmonary embolus**

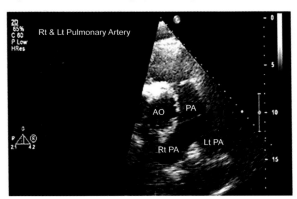

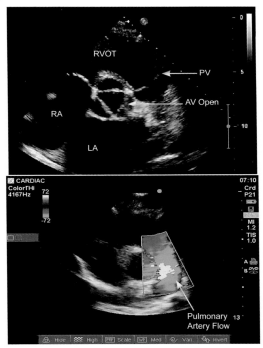

Apical Window / 4 Chamber View

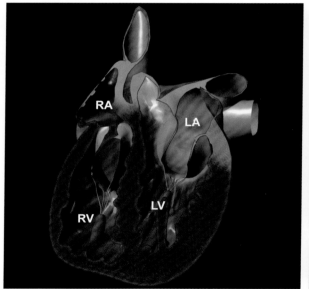

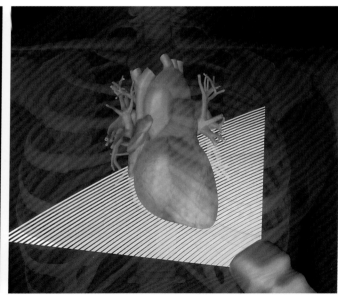

Apical Window/4 Chamber View – Myocardial segments

Transducer Placement

Start location: **C2**

Place the transducer at the apex with the footprint towards the patient's head or right shoulder. Transducer marker is rotated to approximately 3 o'clock position

Sonographic Findings

Examine the **overall cardiac contractility**

Note any wall motion abnormality in different segments

Lateral, Apical, Septal

Can be used to estimate the **EF** – Evaluate the **RV function**

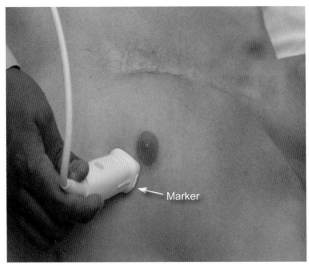

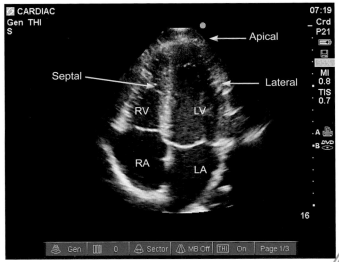

Apical Window/4 Chamber View – MV & TV Function

Sonographic Findings (cont.)

Use CF to examine the MV and TV function and detect any significant **flow** abnormality

Note any significant MV, TV stenosis or regurgitation

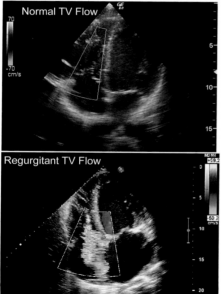

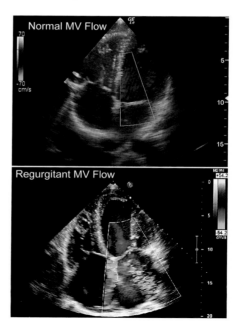

Echo Abnormalities

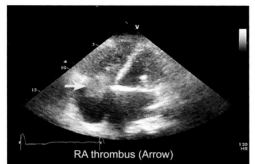

RA thrombus (Arrow)

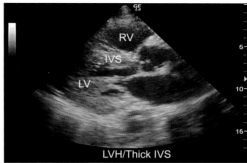

LVH/Thick IVS

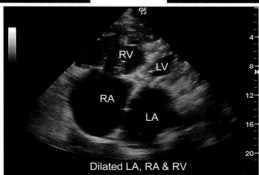

Dilated LA, RA & RV

Apical Window/ 5 Chamber View

Transducer Placement

Start location: **C2**
5 Chamber: Tilting the transducer upward at the apex to open up the **LVOT and Aortic valve** (the 5th chamber)

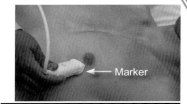
Marker

Sonographic Findings

- Using the **CF** can help identify the 5th chamber
- Using CF and PW Doppler to calculate the stroke volume (SV) as well as any significant regurgitation

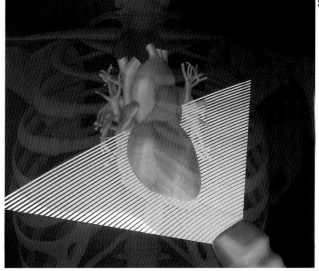

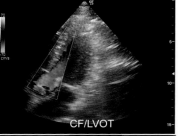
CF/LVOT

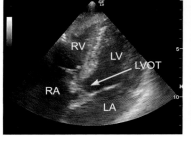
RV LV LVOT RA LA

Apical Window/ 2 Chamber View

Transducer Placement

Start location: **C2**
Rotate the transducer 45° CCW from the 4 Chamber view. Transducer marker at about 12 o'clock

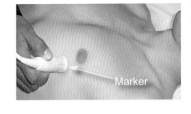

Sonographic Findings

Examine myocardial segments

- Anterior
- Posterior
- Apical

Evaluate MV function and abnormalities

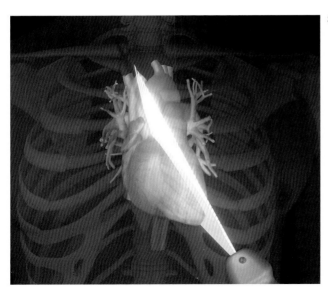

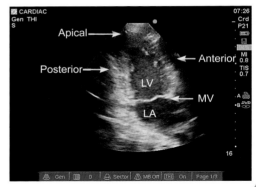

Subcostal Window/4 Chamber View

Transducer Placement

Start location: **C3**

4 Chamber: Below the xiphoid process, the footprint pointing towards the left shoulder. The marker is at about 3 o'clock position

Sonographic Findings

Evaluate the function of all chambers

Note any wall motion abnormality

Good view to detect any pericardial effusion

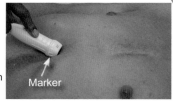

Marker

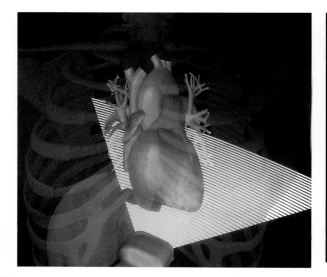

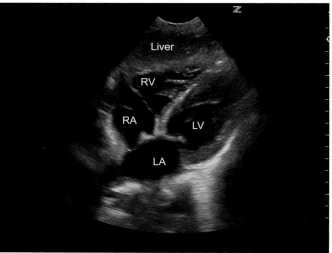

Liver

RV

RA

LV

LA

Subcostal Window/Short axis

Transducer Placement

Start location: **C3**

Short axis: From the 4 chamber view, rotate the transducer 90° CW so that the transducer marker is pointing at about 6 o'clock or 12 o'clock

Sonographic Findings

Similar to the parasternal short axis view

Can show the heart segments at different levels

Used for IVC assessment

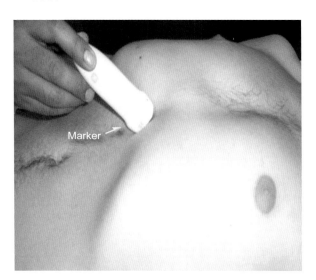

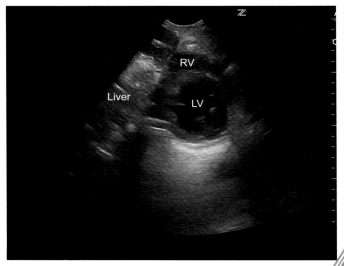

Subcostal/Inferior Vena Cava (IVC)

Transducer Placement

Start location: **C3**

Curvilinear transducer can be used

Depth 15-20 cm

Subcostal, the **footprint pointing towards the spine** and the transducer marker is pointing cephalad

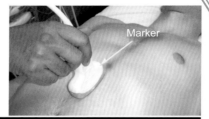

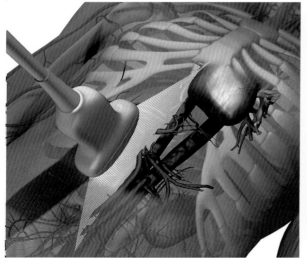

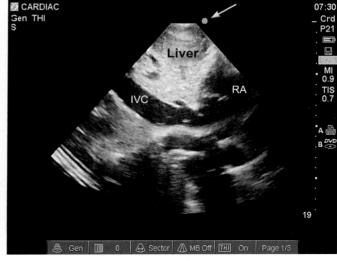

Sonographic Findings (cont.)

To evaluate the **volume status**:
Note the IVC diameter and its changes with the respiratory cycle

Normal IVC diameter is **1.5-2.5 cm** during expiration in a spon-taneously breathing patient, just **distal to the hepatic vein**

Change in IVC diameter is an accurate predictor of fluid respon-siveness

Change in IVC diameter > 50% indicates that the patient is possibly hypovolemic

Change of less than 20%, the patient will probably not respond to fluid challenge

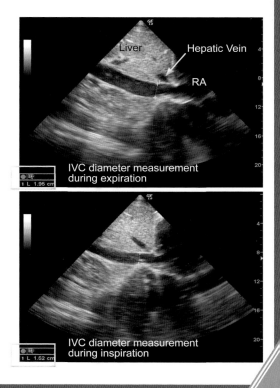

IVC diameter measurement during expiration

IVC diameter measurement during inspiration

Subcostal/IVC

By using the **M Mode**, the IVC diameter measurement is more accurate

Remember that the diameter change during the respiratory cycle is reversed in Mechanically ventilated patients (i.e. Smaller during expiration and larger during inspiration)

Sometimes in quiet respiration, the IVC may not change in diameter. A **"sniff test"** can be done to observe the change

IVC diameter < 1.5 cm and collapsing, indicates hypovolemia.

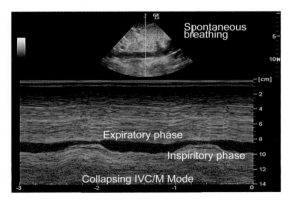

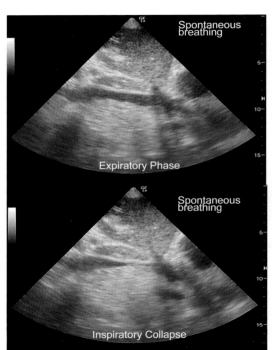

Suprasternal View / Evaluation of Aorta

Transducer Position

Start location: **C4**

Place the transducer in the Suprasternal notch with the footprint pointing towards the back of the sternum. The patient's head is turned to the side

Long axis = Transducer marker at about 2 o'clock

Short axis = Transducer marker at about 5 o'clock

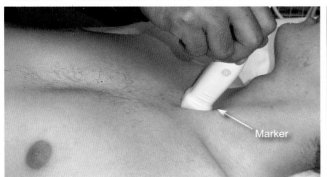

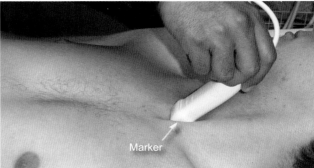

Suprasternal View / Evaluation of Aorta

Sonographic Findings

Long Axis

The ascending aorta, aortic arch, descending aorta, the right pulmonary artery and the brachycephalic vessels will be in view

Examine for the presence of any **dissection or moving flap**

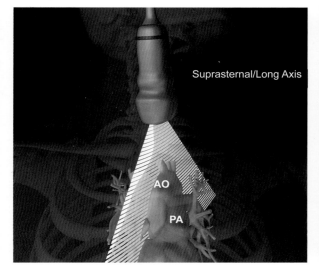

Suprasternal/Long Axis

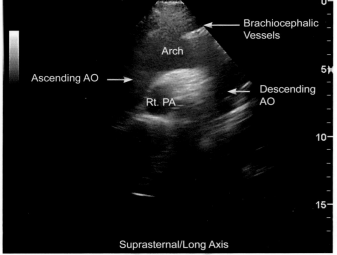

Suprasternal View / Evaluation of Aorta

Sonographic Findings

Short Axis

The aortic arch (in short axis), Superior Vena Cava (SVC) and the right pulmonary artery in its long axis

Examine for the presence of any dissection or moving flap

Use **CF** to help visualize the flow and **false lumen** if present

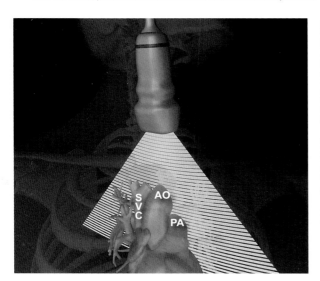

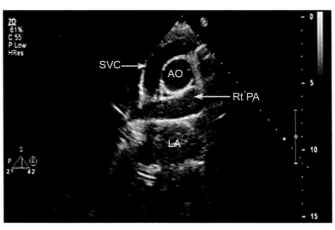

LV Systolic Function Evaluation
Ejection Fraction (EF)

Indications

Useful in managing hypotensive patients

Differentiate cardiogenic from non-cardiogenic shock

LV systolic function can be accurately assessed by critical care physicians using ultrasound in hypotensive patients

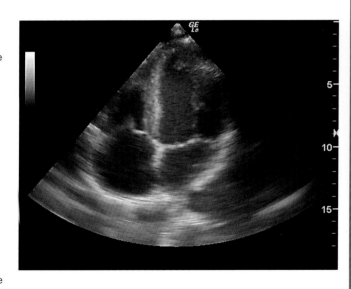

EF can be assessed by:

Simpson's Method or modified Simpson's Method

- Apical 4 chamber and/or 2 chamber view should be obtained
- The software divides the LV volume into 20 slices of equal height
- Volume size=Slice area X Slice thickness
- EF=LVEDV-LVESV/LVEDV X 100%

B Mode (Eyeballing)

Visual estimation of LV EF

M Mode

Software compares LV diameter in systole and end diastole

Normal EF=50-70%

LV Systolic Function Evaluation
EF

EF (cont.)

Simpson's Method Steps

- Acquire an apical 4 chamber and 2 chamber view and store the loops and images
- With the tracking ball, trace the LV cavity at end diastole, and then at end systole for both the 4 and 2 chamber views

EF=LVEDV-LVESV/LVEDV X 100%

Cardiac package will calculate the average results

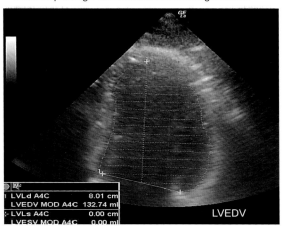

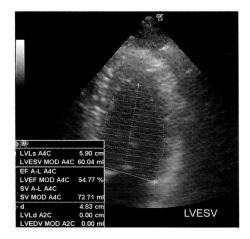

LV Systolic Function Evaluation
Eyeballing

EF (cont.)

Eyeballing, in the experienced eye, is as accurate as formal measurements
Best to obtain a parasternal short axis view at the **papillary muscle level**, or an Apical 4 chamber view and estimate the EF

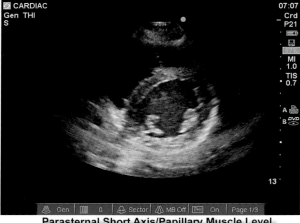

Parasternal Short Axis/Papillary Muscle Level

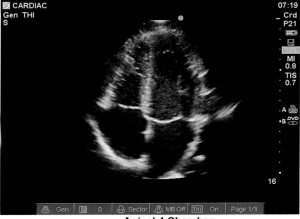

Apical 4 Chamber

LV systolic Function Evaluation
EF

EF (cont.)

M Mode

Measure the **LVIDd** (LV internal dimension end diastole)
- LVIDd range about 3.5-6.5 cm

Measure the **LVIDs** (LV internal diameter end systole)
- LVIDs range about 2.0-3.8 cm

Cardiac package will calculate the EF & SV as well as fractional shortening

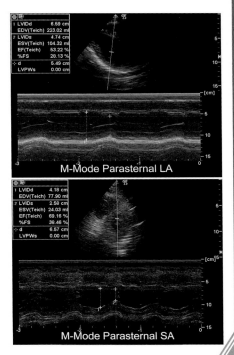

M-Mode Parasternal LA

M-Mode Parasternal SA

LV Systolic Function Evaluation
Stroke Volume (SV)

SV Measurement

Simpson's Method or modified Simpson's will be used

Simpson's Method Steps

- Acquire an apical 4 chamber and 2 chamber view

- With the track ball, trace the LV cavity at end diastole, and then at end systole for both the 4 and 2 chamber views

SV= LVEDV-LVESV
Normal= 60-70 ml

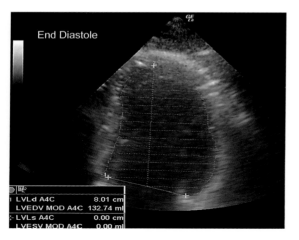

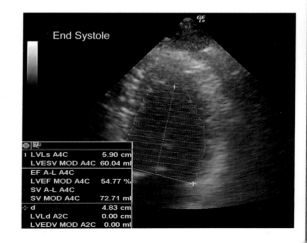

LV systolic Function Evaluation
SV Measurement

SV Measurement (cont.)
Aortic Root method (2 steps)

Measure **diameter** of the aorta by M Mode or 2 D Echo

- CSA (Cross Sectional Area) = 2 (Diameter)² X 0.78
- Normal CSA 1.8-2.2 cm

Measure flow velocity, **VTI** (Velocity Time Index) from the
LVOT at peak systole by PW Doppler

Calculate the volume of flow (SV)

- SV= Cross sectional area X Velocity
- **SV= CSA X VTI**
- Cardiac package will do calculations

How to obtain VTI

Remember that the transducer angle is critical

Obtain a 5 chamber apical view

Use CF to help identify the 5th chamber (LVOT)

Use PW Doppler and point the marker to the LVOT

Using the track ball, track the systolic Doppler wave

Velocity of flow from the LVOT at peak systole by 2D echo
(VTI) will be calculated by the cardiac package

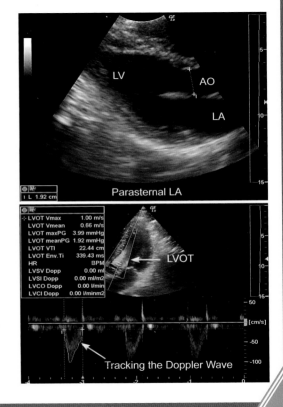

Parasternal LA

LVOT Vmax	1.00 m/s
LVOT Vmean	0.66 m/s
LVOT maxPG	3.99 mmHg
LVOT meanPG	1.92 mmHg
LVOT VTI	22.44 cm
LVOT Env.Ti	339.43 ms
HR	BPM
LVSV Dopp	0.00 ml
LVSI Dopp	0.00 ml/m2
LVCO Dopp	0.00 l/min
LVCI Dopp	0.00 l/minm2

LVOT

Tracking the Doppler Wave

Right Heart Assessment

Transducer Placement
The right heart can be assessed through different windows, **C1,C2 and C3**

Start location: **C1**

From the parasternal long axis view of the LV, tilt the transducer with the footprint pointing slightly towards the right thigh

RV assessment
Examine the RV inflow tract **(RVIT)** and any significant TV regurgitation

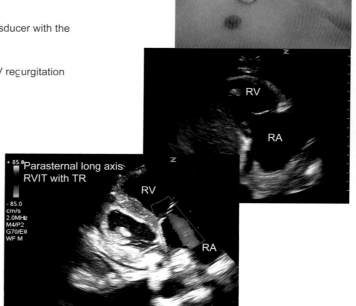

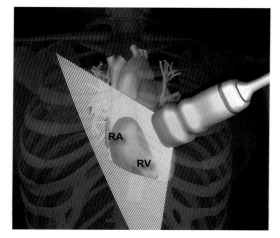

Right Heart Assessment

Sonographic Findings

C3/Subcostal

- Examine the **wall motion and contractility**, any paradoxical septal movement
- EF in RV is normally less than LV
- RVED area is usually **< 2/3** of the LVED area
- Note any RV dilation or collapse
- Good view to detect any **pericardial effusion**

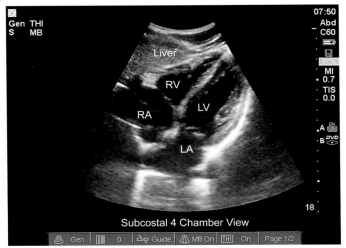

Subcostal 4 Chamber View

Pulmonary Artery Pressure (PAP) Assessment

Transducer Placement

C2/Apical 4 chamber view

Sonographic Findings/Steps

Assuming **TR** is present in most patients (over 75% of normal adults)

Turn color flow and continuous wave Doppler across the Tricuspid valve

Align cursor along TV regurgitation jet when noted

Mark the maximum TR jet

- Normal TR Velocity is 1.7-2.3 m/s
- The signal reflects the pressure gradient between RV and RA
- A higher velocity usually means a higher PAP

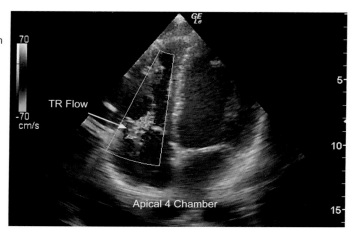

TR Flow

Apical 4 Chamber

PAP Assessment

Sonographic Findings/Steps (cont.)

PA pressure = 4 X (peak TR velocity)^2 + RA pressure (usually 5-10 mmHg)

RA pressure or CVP can be estimated from
- Jugular Venous Pressure
- Respiratory variation of the IVC

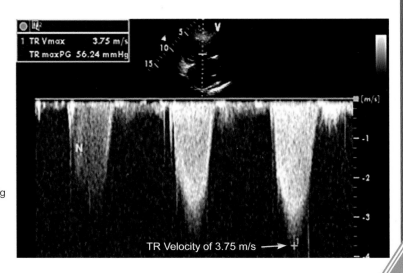

Example:

If peak TR velocity is 3.75 m/s
and the estimated RA pressure is 10 mmHg

PA pressure = 4 X (3.75)^2 + 10 = 66.25 mmHg

Pulmonary Artery End Diastolic Pressure (PAEDP) Assessment/ Wedge Pressure

Transducer Placement

Start Location: **C1**/Left Parasternal Short axis View of the **RVOT**. Apply continuous Doppler

Sonographic Findings

- Pulmonary Incompetence is common
- **PAEDP**=4 X(Pulmonary Regurgitation End Diastolic Velocity PREDV)^2 + RAP
- Estimation of the RAP is as mentioned before

Example (below):
If PAREDV was 2 m/s and RAP was 10 then
PAEDP= 4 X $(2)^2$ + 10= 26 mmHg

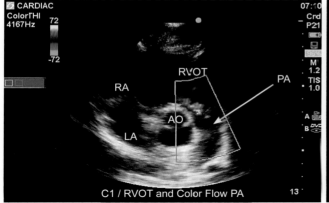

C1 / RVOT and Color Flow PA

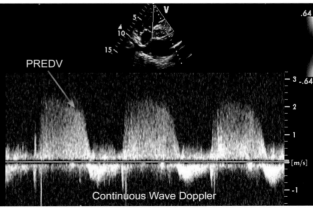

Continuous Wave Doppler

Pericardial Effusion

Transducer Placement

C3/Subcostal/The better view
C1/Parasternal
C2/Apical

Sonographic Findings

C3/Subcostal

Detection of echo-free rim around the heart within the hyperechoic parietal pericardium

False positive

- Pleural effusion
- Epicardial fat pad (usually anterior)

Measure the pericardial space in systole and diastole

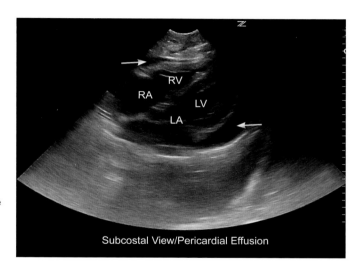

Subcostal View/Pericardial Effusion

Pericardial Effusion

Sonographic Findings (cont.)

C1/Parasternal View

- A pericardial effusion will accumulate between the heart and the descending aorta.
- A pleural effusion will accumulate beyond the descending aorta and will not separate it from the heart
- Physiological effusion measures < 1 cm and is posterior only
- Moderate is < 1 cm and large is > 1 cm in measurement and circumferential

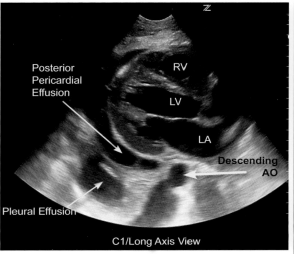

C1/Long Axis View

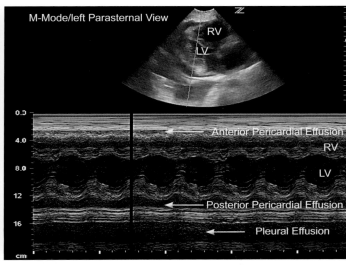

Cardiac Tamponade

Transducer Placement

Start location: **C3**/ Subcostal

Sonographic Findings

RA and RV **diastolic collapse**

RV free wall moves towards the RV cavity early in diastole [normally it moves away]

RA moves inwards at the end of diastole and the beginning of systole.

Small amounts of pericardial effusion, when accumulating acutely, can lead to Tamponade features

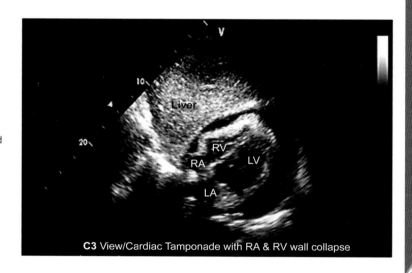

C3 View/Cardiac Tamponade with RA & RV wall collapse

Cardiac Tamponade

Sonographic Findings (cont.)

Obtaining an **M-Mode** with the cursor across the RV free wall, will show the collapse

Preserved reactivity of the IVC (changing with the respiratory cycle), strongly argues against hemodynamically significant cardiac Tamponade.

This can be examined by the IVC 2D or M-Mode images

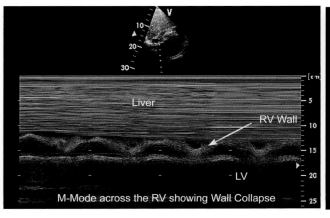

M-Mode across the RV showing Wall Collapse

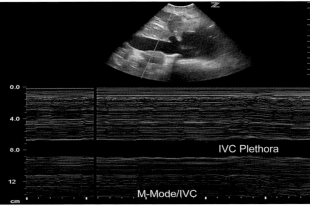

M-Mode/IVC

Cardiac Tamponade

Sonographic Findings

The heart will display a **"swinging motion"**, which is an ominous sign of cardiac tamponade

By applying the Doppler, MV and TV flows will show exaggerated velocity features with respiration

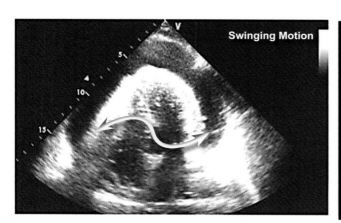

Swinging Motion

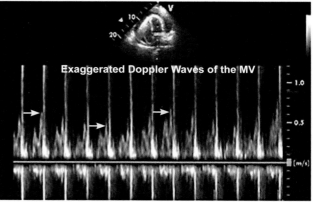

Exaggerated Doppler Waves of the MV

Cardiac Arrest

Echocardiography can be performed during cardiac arrest and CPR

Helps detect cardiac motion, dilated RV, pericardial effusion, cardiac tamponade and PEA

An image of the heart can be obtained in **C3** (Subxiphiod 4 chamber) or **C1** (Left parasternal long axis)

View Cardiac contractility and wall motion

Detect any **intra-cardiac thrombi** (associated with poor prognosis)

Exam should be done during pulse checks, lasting no more than 5-7 seconds

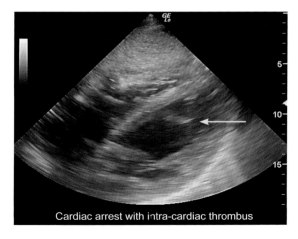

Cardiac arrest with intra-cardiac thrombus

Worksheet

Patient Name: _____

MRN: _____

Date: _____

Echo Performer: _____

LV & LA

Global LV Size	Normal ☐	Dilated ☐
Wall Motion Abnormality	Y ☐	N ☐
Segment	_____	
LA	Normal ☐	Dilated ☐
LV Function (EF)	>40% ☐ <40% ☐	_____ %

RV & RA

Global LV Size	Normal ☐	Dilated ☐
RVEDA/LVEDA	0.6-1 ☐	>1 ☐
Paradoxical Septal Motion	Y ☐	N ☐
Dilated RA	Y ☐	

Valve Abnormality (Moderate-Severe)

	Y ☐	N ☐
MVR	Y ☐	N ☐
AVR	Y ☐	N ☐
TVR	Y ☐	N ☐
PVR	Y ☐	N ☐

Pericardial Effusion

	Y ☐	N ☐
Small <1 cm Posterior only	Y ☐	N ☐
Moderate <1 cm circumferencial	Y ☐	N ☐
Large >1 cm circumferential	Y ☐	N ☐

Tamponade

	Y ☐	N ☐
RA/RV collapse	Y ☐	N ☐
Dilated non-collapsible IVC (IVC Plethora)	Y ☐	N ☐

IVC Size and Collapsibility Index

	Y ☐	N ☐
< 1.5 cm & collapse	Y ☐	N ☐
1.5-2.5 cm	Y ☐	N ☐
>2.5 cm	Y ☐	N ☐
>50% diameter change	Y ☐	N ☐
<50% diameter change	Y ☐	N ☐
Estimated RAP (CVP)	_____	

Aortic Dissection

	Y ☐	N ☐
Intimal Flap	Y ☐	N ☐
Pericardial Effusion	Y ☐	N ☐
Aortic Regurgitation	Y ☐	N ☐

Cardiac Arrest

	Y ☐	N ☐
Cardiac Standstill	Y ☐	N ☐
Pericardial Tamponade	Y ☐	N ☐
Intracardiac Thrombus	Y ☐	N ☐
Dilated RV & RA	Y ☐	N ☐

Impressions, Comments and Recommendations

Abdominal Exam

J. Antonio Bouffard, MD
Patrick R. Meyers, BS, RDMS

Contents

* Focused Assessment with Sonography for Trauma

Abdominal Exam

Transducer Placement

Views may vary with anatomy,
type of injury, body habitus and position

- **A1**: Subxiphoid
    - Cardiac, IVC, Aorta
- **A2**: Right or Left Subcostal, mid-clavicular line
    - IVC, Aorta
- **A3**: Right or Left Subcostal, Anterior Axillary line
    - Liver, GB, spleen
- **A4**: Right or Left mid to posterior Axillay line at the level of 7th Intercostal space to the flank area
    - Bowel,Liver, Spleen, Kidney, Diaphragm,
- **A5**: Right or Left 7th -10th intercostal space anterior axillary line
    - Liver, GB, Spleen, Lung, heart
- **A6**: Abdominal Midline
    - Aorta, IVC, Pancreas
- **A7**: Suprapubic
    - Bladder
    - Uterus

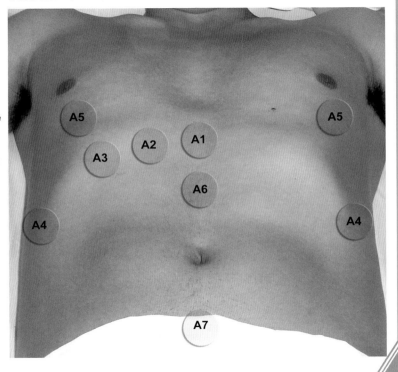

Abdominal Exam

Transducer Type & Orientation

Curvilinear transducer, 2 - 5 MHz or a phased array transducer

Transducer marker pointing cephalad (for sagittal plane) or towards the patient's right (for transverse plane)

Screen marker on the left side of the screen

Depth about 15-20 cm

Patient Position

Supine

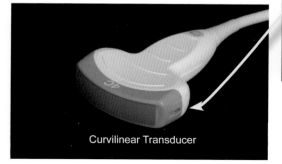

Curvilinear Transducer

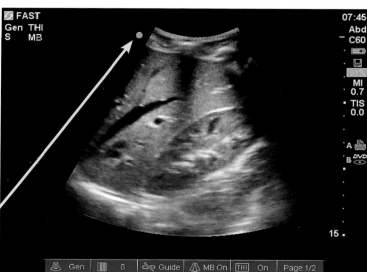

FAST Exam

Transducer Placement

A1 Subxiphoid view/Pericardial

A4 RUQ/Hepatorenal recess (Morrison's pouch)

A4 LUQ/Splenorenal recess

A7 Suprapubic/Pelvic

FAST exam results should only complement the clinical exam and other diagnostic modalities to reach a final decision

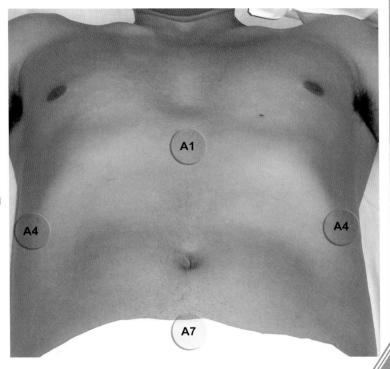

FAST/Sub-xiphoid view

Patient position
Supine

Transducer Placement
A1 Subxiphoid, pointing towards the left shoulder with the transducer marker pointing towards the patient's right

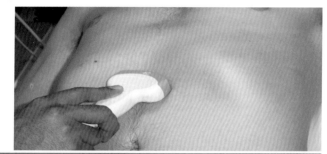

Structures to be identified
Heart
Liver
IVC

Sonographic Findings
Able to detect any significant pericardial effusion or Tamponade

- Pericardium is hyperechoic

- The pericardial space is anechoic or hypoechoic space between the heart and Pericardium

- Normally, minimal pericardial fluid is present

- False positive: pleural effusion and epicardial fat pad

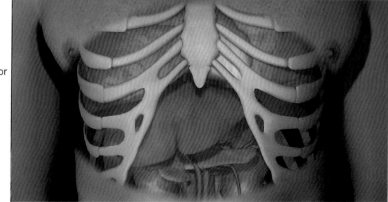

FAST/Sub-xiphoid view

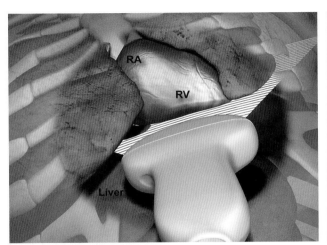

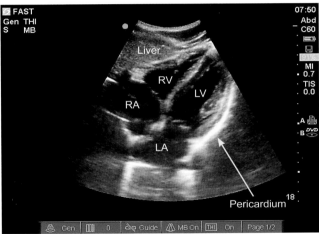

FAST/Sub-xiphoid view

Sonographic Findings (cont.)

Acute minimal fluid accumulations can lead to hemodynamic compromise

Assess the general cardiac function

Evaluate

- RV function

- RA collapse (in the case of Tamponade)

- IVC diameter and respiratory variation to determine the effect of the pericardial effusion on the cardiac function (Discussed later in the chapter)

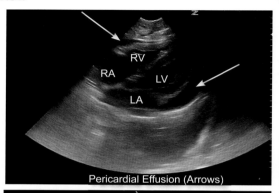

Pericardial Effusion (Arrows)

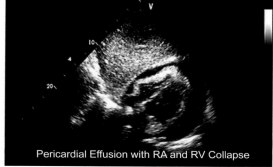

Pericardial Effusion with RA and RV Collapse

FAST/RUQ/Hepatorenal Recess (Morrison's View)

Patient position
- Supine
- Trendelenburg position may give a better view of the RUQ structures

Transducer Placement
- **A3** Right subcostal, anterior axillary line
- **A4** About mid axillary line, 7th intercostal space to the right flank area
- Marker cephalad
- **A4 CCW** rotation and oblique positioning will help eliminate the rib shadows
- Angle of the transducer can be moved more cephalad to examine the lungs and pleura

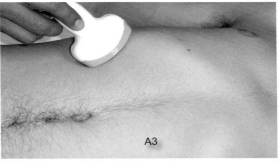
A3

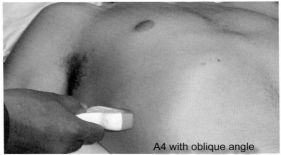
A4 with oblique angle

FAST/RUQ/Hepatorenal Recess(Morrison's View)

Structures to be identified

Liver
Diaphragm
Kidney
Morrison's Pouch

Sonographic Findings

- Hepatorenal recess **(Morrison's Pouch)** Found more posteriorly

- Sliding the transducer downward will expose the lower edge of the liver where free fluid tends to accumulate

- Sliding the transducer upward will expose the right diaphragm, pleural space and lungs

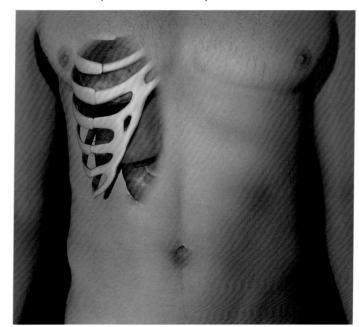

FAST/RUQ/Hepatorenal Recess(Morrison's View)

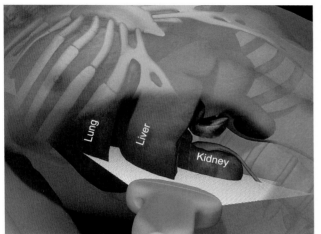
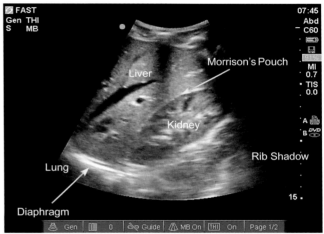

FAST/RUQ/Hepatorenal Recess(Morrison's View)

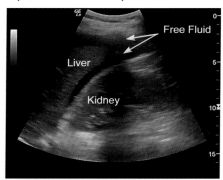

Sonographic Findings (cont.)

The RUQ is the most common location to identify intra-abdominal free fluid or blood

Anechoic or hypoechoic space between the liver and kidney indicates free fluid, which also tends to accumulate in the subdiaphragmatic region or near the inferior pole of the kidney

Measure the width of the anechoic stripe in Morrison's pouch

Width in **cm**= Abdominal fluid in **Liters**

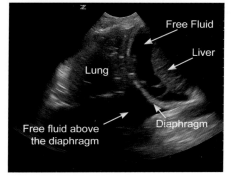

FAST/LUQ/Perisplenic

Patient position
- Supine

Transducer Placement
- **A3** Left subcostal, anterior axillary line
- **A4** About the mid – posterior axillary line, 7th intercostal space - left flank area
- Marker cephalad
- Oblique Position with **CW** rotation can help eliminate the rib shadows

Structures to be identified
Spleen
Kidney
Lung, Diaphragm
Splenorenal Recess

Sonographic Findings
- Locate the splenorenal recess
- Sliding the transducer downward will expose the lower tip of the spleen where free fluid tends to accumulate
- Sliding the transducer upward will expose the left diaphragm and pleural space

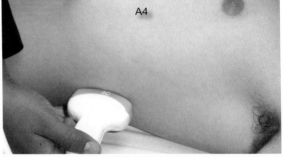

A4

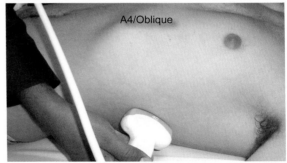

A4/Oblique

FAST/LUQ/Perisplenic

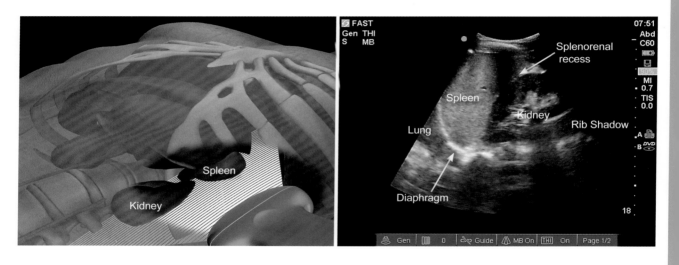

Sonographic Findings (cont.)

Fluid can collect between the diaphragm and the spleen in the left upper quadrant.

Fluid will present as hypoechoic or anechoic strip

- Measure the width of the anechoic stripe

    Width in **cm**= Abdominal fluid in **Liters**

- Hemothorax will present as a hypoechoic strip above the diaphragm

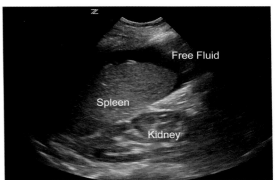

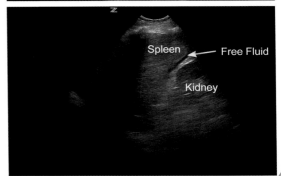

FAST/Suprapubic

Patient position

- Supine

Transducer Placement

A7 Above pubis angled inferiorly

Obtain both the transverse and longitudinal views

- **Transverse View:**
  marker pointing towards the patient's right

- **Longitudinal view:**
  marker pointing cephalad

Structures to be identified

Bladder

Uterus (if applicable)

Prostate (if applicable)

Cul De Sac

Retrovesical space

Sonographic Findings

- Better to perform the US on a full bladder

- Obtain a long and short axis views

- Accumulated free fluid will be found as a hypoechoic strip in the **cul de sac** or **retrovesicular** space on either side of the bladder

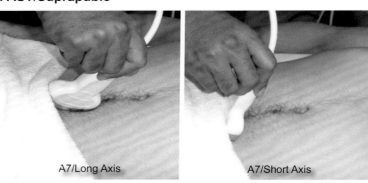

A7/Long Axis   A7/Short Axis

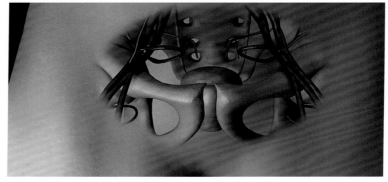

FAST/Suprapubic

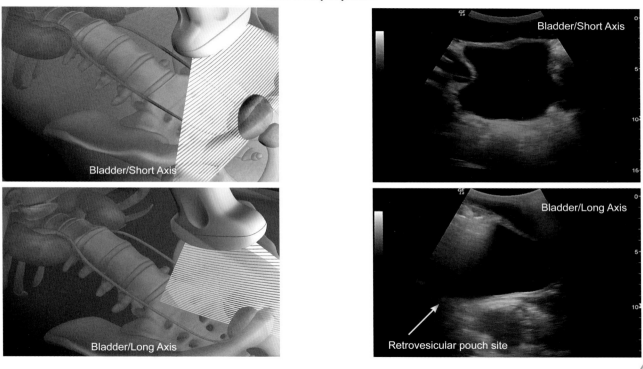

Bladder/Short Axis

Bladder/Long Axis

Bladder/Short Axis

Bladder/Long Axis

Retrovesicular pouch site

FAST/Suprapubic

Sonographic Findings (cont.)

Less than 20 ml of fluid is considered normal in an adult.

Bladder volume measurement can be estimated:

- Height X Width X Depth X 0.5
- By measuring the long and short axis, the ultrasound software will estimate the volume
- Normal Measurements
- Long axis: 10-12 cm
- Short axis: 5 cm
- Normal bladder wall thickness is 5 mm when empty and 3 mm when full

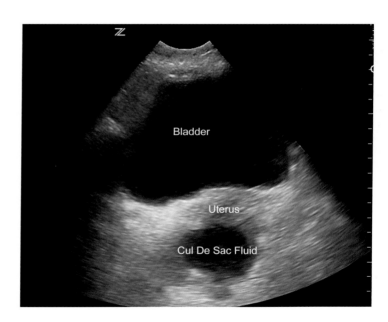

Extended FAST (E-FAST) Examination

Extended FAST

Lungs & Pleural interface

To detect the presence of pneumothorax or pleural effusion

IVC

To evaluate the fluid status and guide resuscitation efforts

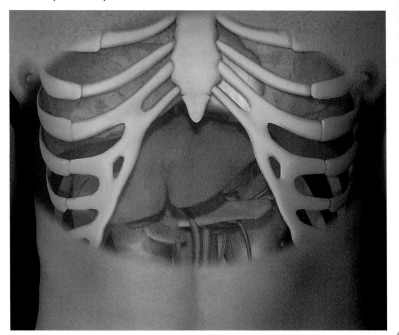

PREFACE
FOREWORD
GETTING
STARTED
CARDIAC ABDOMINAL AORTA VASCULAR LUNG OPTIC
NERVE
OB/GYN SOFT TISSUE
BONE & DVT
PROCEDURES PROTOCOLS 87

E-FAST/Lung

Extended FAST (cont.)

Patient position

- Supine

Transducer Type & Placement

- Phased array 2.5-5 MHz or Linear 7-13 MHz

- Curvilinear 2-5 MHz for deeper penetration

- **L1**, 2nd-4th intercostal spaces, anterior chest wall

- **L2**, 5th-8th intercostal spaces, anterior chest wall

- **L3**, 4th-10th intercostal spaces, between the anterior & posterior axillary lines

Transducer Placement

Transducer marker pointing cephalad

The exam should be performed bilaterally

Depth about 15-20 cm

Structures to be identified

Lungs

Diaphragm

Liver & Spleen

Pleural interface

Ribs

Pleural fluid and pneumothorax if present

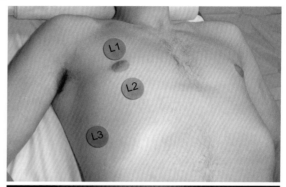

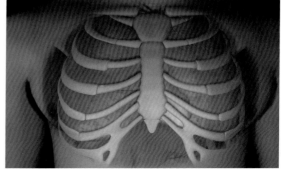

E-FAST Exam/Lung

Sonographic Findings

First, identify the lung, the diaphragm and the liver interface

* Sliding the transducer downward in **L3** can give a good view of the lungs and diaphragm

Look for normal and abnormal lung signs

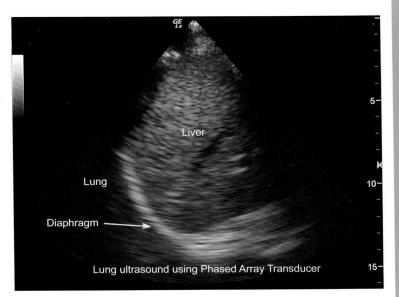

Lung ultrasound using Phased Array Transducer

E-FAST Exam/Lung

Sonographic Findings (cont.)

"Lung Sliding" Sign/Normal

- Two echogenic pleural lines sliding with respiration and heart motion. Tend to be slightly hyperechoic. Best in **L1 & L2**

- Color Flow (CF) can help identify lung sliding. Color will be present at the pleural interface with respiration

- The presence of lung sliding rules out pneumothorax

- Perform the US exam bilaterally in **L1, L2 and L3**

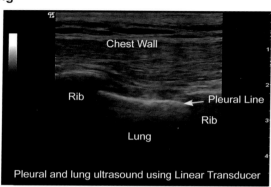

Pleural and lung ultrasound using Linear Transducer

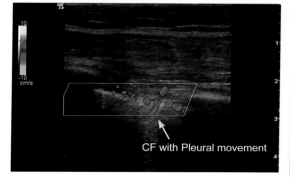

CF with Pleural movement

Sonographic Findings (cont.)

Seashore Sign (sand on the beach)/Normal

- Start with the **B Mode** and identify the lung sliding
- Switch to **M-Mode** and place the cursor on the pleural line
  - The soft tissue and the pleural structures will appear as horizontal lines.
- The presence of the seashore sign rules out pneumothorax

Pneumothorax

No "Lung Sliding" Sign

- Air will prevent the visceral pleura from being visualized, and the sliding motion will not be seen
- No color will be present at the pleural interface when CF is applied

M-Mode

- **Stratosphere Sign**/sand on the beach is not seen.

Perform the US exam bilaterally and in all lung areas

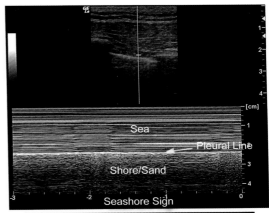

Seashore Sign

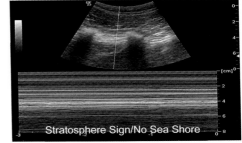

Stratosphere Sign/No Sea Shore

E-FAST Exam/Lung

Sonographic Findings (cont.)

Pleural Effusion

Best detected in **L3** area in a supine patient

Anechoic space separating the parietal and visceral pleura

Note the lung movement with respiration **(Jelly Fish Sign)**

Fluid Volume

- Measure the fluid depth at the lung base or the level of the 5th intercostal space
- Measurement starts approximately 3 cm from the inferior pole of the lung to the chest wall
- **> 5 cm** fluid thickness indicate pleural effusion **> 500 ml**

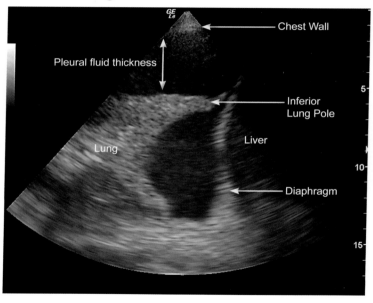

E-FAST/Inferior Vena Cava (IVC)

E-FAST (cont.)

Patient position
- Supine

Transducer
- Curvilinear 2-5 MHz or Phased Array 2.5-5 MHz

Transducer Position
- **A2, A1**
- Marker Cephalad

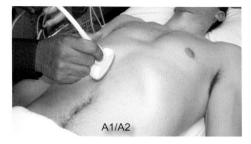

A1/A2

Structures to be identified
IVC

Right Atrium

Liver

Hepatic veins

Aorta

Sonographic findings
Start from A1 or A2 position and slide the transducer towards the patient's right

Identify the IVC, right atrium and the liver

Make sure to differentiate the IVC from the Aorta, which has thicker walls, gives the SMA and celiac branches and is pulsatile

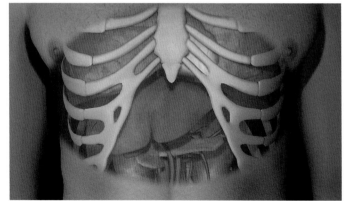

E-FAST Exam/IVC

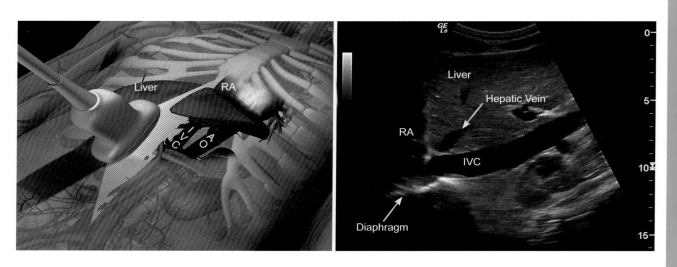

E-FAST Exam/IVC

Sonographic Findings (cont.)

To evaluate the **volume status**

- The IVC diameter changes during the respiratory cycle, smaller during inspiration, larger during expiration. In mechanically ventilated patients, this relationship is reversed

- In the case of RVF/ RV infarct, massive PE, TR or cardiac Tamponade, there will be a distended IVC, and no variation with respiration (IVC Plethora)

During spontaneous breathing, the normal IVC diameter is **1.5-2.5 cm** during expiration, just distal to the hepatic vein

Small IVC diameter and > 50% change during respiration usually indicate hypovolemia

Less than 20% change during respiration, the patient probably will not respond to fluid challenge

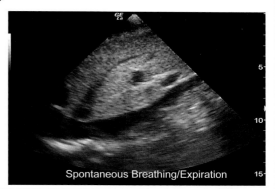
Spontaneous Breathing/Expiration

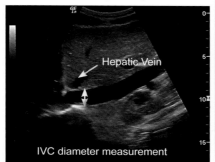
Hepatic Vein

IVC diameter measurement

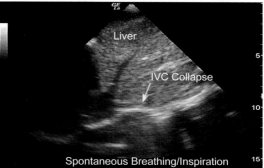
Liver

IVC Collapse

Spontaneous Breathing/Inspiration

E-FAST/IVC

By using the **M Mode**, the IVC diameter measurement is more accurate

IVC diameter change during the respiratory cycle is **reversed** in mechanically ventilated patients
(i.e. smaller in expiration and larger during inspiration)

Sometimes in quiet respiration, the IVC may not change in diameter. A **"sniff test"** can help observe the change

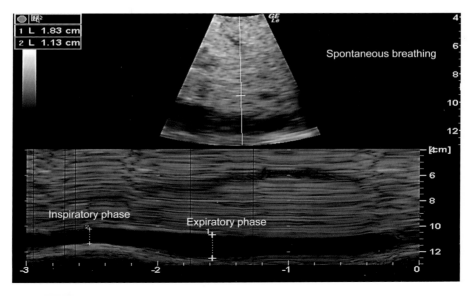

Gallbladder (GB) & Common Bile Duct (CBD)

Indications
Right upper quadrant or epigastric pain

Suspicion of cholecystitis, cholangitis

Patient Position
Supine

>Deep breath can help push the GB down

>Left lateral decubitus helps bring the gallbladder out from beneath the ribs

>The GB is not a fixed organ and its position can vary

Transducer type & Placement
Curvilinear 2-5 MHz or Phased Array 2.5-5 MHz

A3, A5

Long Axis
Marker pointing cephalad

Short Axis
Marker pointing towards the patient's right

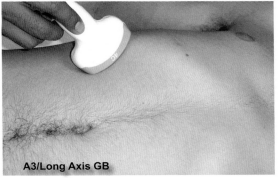

A3/Long Axis GB

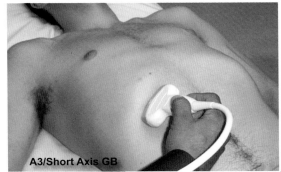

A3/Short Axis GB

GB & CBD

Structures to be identified

GB

Liver

CBD

Portal Vein, Hepatic artery, IVC

Sonographic Findings

- The GB is generally found between the nipple line and anterior axillary line

- Scan the inferior edge of the liver, medial to the kidney, and lateral to the IVC

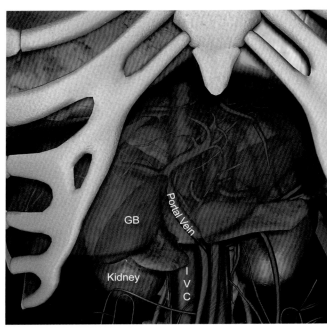

GB & CBD

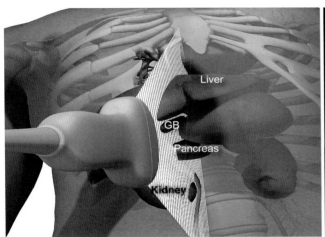

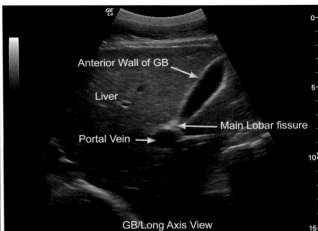

Liver

GB

Pancreas

Kidney

Anterior Wall of GB

Liver

Main Lobar fissure

Portal Vein

GB/Long Axis View

GB & CBD

Sonographic Findings (cont.)

Long Axis/GB
Transduceer Placement

Start with the transducer at **A3** with the marker cephalad, may need to go to **A5** with the marker towards the right axilla (transhepatic)

Scan the entire GB from the neck to the fundus by panning the transducer

The main lobar fissure connects the Portal vein to the bladder neck

Adding CF will help identify blood vessels. GB has no flow

Note the presence of any sludge or stones

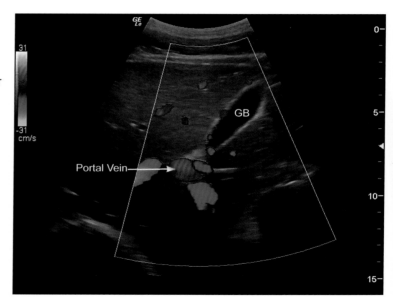

GB & CBD

Sonographic findings (cont.)

Short Axis/GB
Transducer Placement

A3 or A5 From the Long Axis view rotate the transducer CCW so the marker is pointed towards the patient's right or Right Axilla

In many instances the position of the transducer may vary with the anatomy

Tilt the transducer from **cephalad to caudal** orientation to visualize the fundus of the gallbladder to the neck toward the portal triad

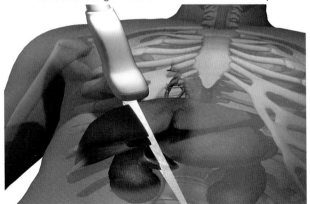

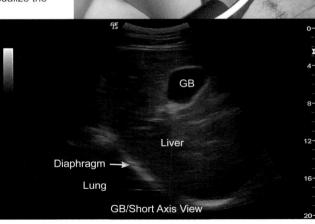

GB

Liver

Diaphragm →

Lung

GB/Short Axis View

GB & CBD

Sonographic Findings (cont.)

Anterior wall thickness measurement

- From the middle of the anterior wall
- Inner to outer surface measurement
- Normal **<3 mm**

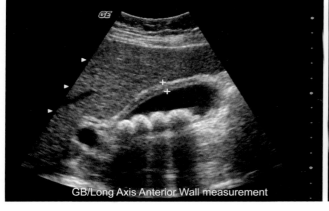

GB/Long Axis Anterior Wall measurement

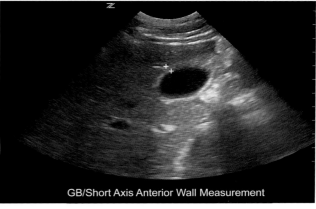

GB/Short Axis Anterior Wall Measurement

Sonographic Findings (cont.)

Cholecystitis/Gall Stones

Thickened anterior wall **> 4 mm**
  • Measurement is taken (in a long and short axis) from the outer to the inner surface.
Presence of **pericholecystic fluid**

Sonographic Murphy's sign

  • Pushing on the GB while in view by US will produce pain
Note the presence of any **stones or sludge**

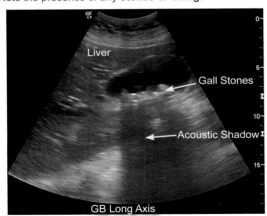

GB Long Axis

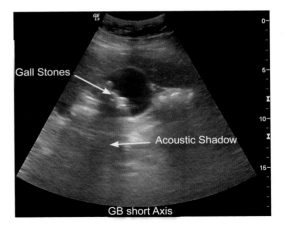

GB short Axis

CHD & CBD

Transducer Placement
A3

Sonographic Findings

- More difficult to detect

- From the long axis view of the GB, follow the anterior wall medially and try to find the connection to the CHD

- Locate the portal vein at the neck of the gallbladder. The CHD is part of the portal triad along with the portal vein and the hepatic artery.

- Rotate the transducer 90° CCW into a longitudinal axis view of the portal vein

- The CBD is found anterior and parallel to the portal vein. Sliding the transducer medially can help identify the CBD.

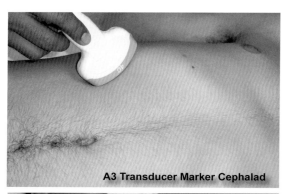

A3 Transducer Marker Cephalad

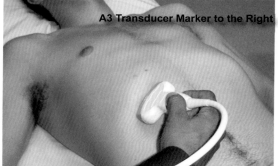

A3 Transducer Marker to the Right

CHD & CBD

Sonographic Findings (cont.)

Long Axis/GB

- CF can help identify the blood vessels. CBD has no flow

- Normal CBD Diameter is less than **7 mm**

- Measurement is between the **interior walls**

- Normal size increases with age and in patients with cholecystectomy

- CBD >10 mm is usually pathologic

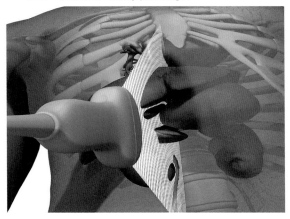

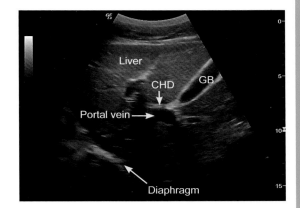

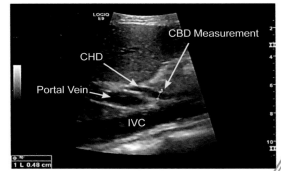

Pancreas

Patient Position

Supine

Transducer Type and Placement

Curvilinear 2-5 MHz

Depth 12-15 cm

Long Axis

A6

Transducer marker towards the patient's right

Short Axis

A6

Transducer marker cephalad

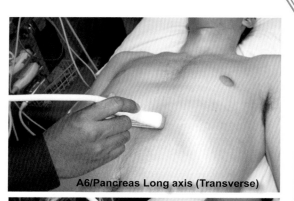

A6/Pancreas Long axis (Transverse)

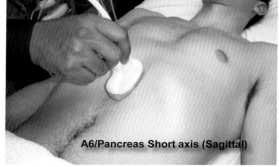

A6/Pancreas Short axis (Sagittal)

Pancreas

Structures to be identified
Pancreas
Aorta
IVC
Splenic Vein
SMA
Spine

Sonographic Findings

The pancreas is found anterior to the splenic vein with homogenous texture

The pancreatic head is anterior to the IVC

The body is parallel to the splenic vein

Pancreatic duct can be visualized horizontally within the gland

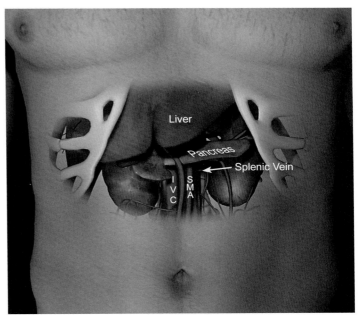

Pancreas

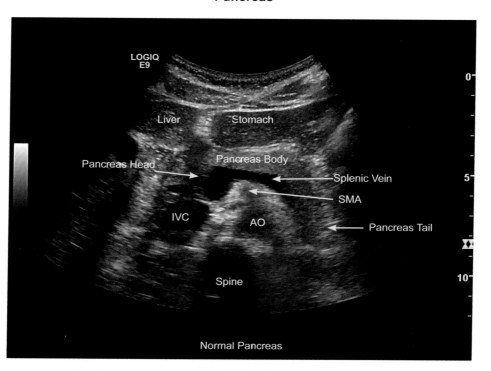

Normal Pancreas

Pancreas

Sonographic Findings (cont.)

Pancreatitis

- The pancreas is larger with a **distorted heterogeneous** pattern. Decrease echogenicity means interstitial edema
- Maximal normal cross section measurements are, head= 2.6 cm and body 2.2 cm
- **Necrotic** area can be identified usually as a hypo-echoic area
- Fluid collection may be found within or outside the pancreas

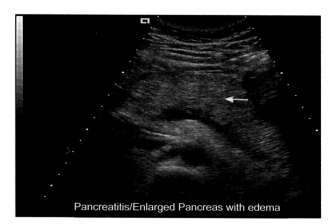

Pancreatitis/Enlarged Pancreas with edema

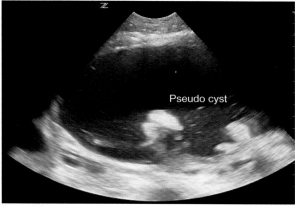

Pseudo cyst

Enlarged Pancreas with a heterogeneous necrotizing pattern

Renal

Indications

Evaluation of acute flank or abdominal pain

To rule out bilateral obstruction in acute renal failure

To evaluate for the presence of stones

To evaluate the bladder

Transducer type and Placement

Curvilinear 2-5 MHz or Phased Array 2.5-5 MHz

A4, A3

Long Axis: Marker pointing cephalad towards the posterior axilla

> May need to slide the transducer from A3 to A4 to the posterior axillary line to obtain a good view

Short Axis: 90° CCW rotation

Patient Position

Supine. Right and left lateral decubitus for left and right kidneys respectively, when possible

A deep breath helps the kidney move below the ribs

Structures to be identified

Kidneys

Liver, Spleen & Diaphragm

Morrison's Pouch and splenorenal recess

Kidney border, Calyces and renal pelvis

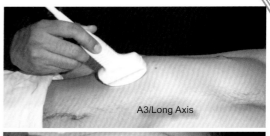

A3/Long Axis

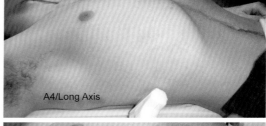

A4/Long Axis

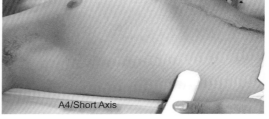

A4/Short Axis

Renal

Transducer Placement/Right kidney
Long Axis

A4, Right mid axillary line from the 7th intercostal space to the right flank with the marker pointing cephalad

Adjust the transducer according to the kidney's long axis (turn CCW) towards the posterior axilla

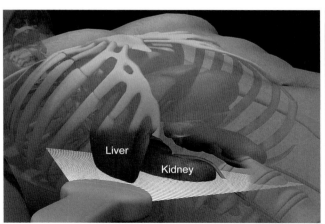

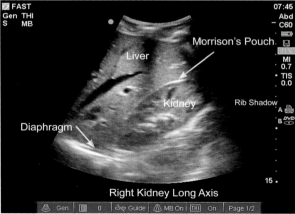

Renal

Transducer Placement/left kidney

Long Axis

A4, Left mid axillary line from the 7th intercostal space to the left flank with the marker pointing cephalad

Adjust the transducer according to the kidney's long axis (turn CW)

More difficult to obtain images compared to the right kidney

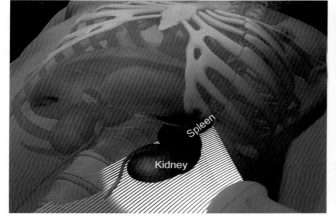

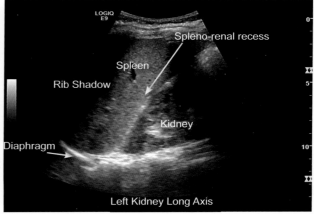

Left Kidney Long Axis

Renal

Transducer Placement

Short Axis

Rotate the transducer 90° counter CCW from the long axis position (either kidney) and tilt the transducer up and down

Sonographic findings

The outer hypoechoic layer consists of the cortex and medulla

The inner layer which is comparatively more echoic consists of the calyces, arteries, veins and the renal pelvis

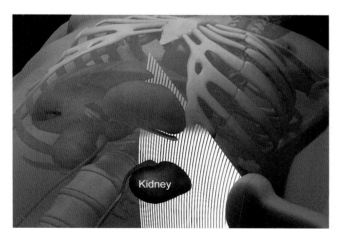

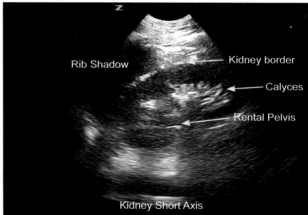

Renal

Sonographic Findings (cont.)

Hydronephrosis

Divided into Grades 1, 2 and 3 depending on the calyceal separation and involvement of the renal pelvis

Normal kidney measurements are length 9-12 cm, and width 4-6 cm

Renal stones appear as hyperechoic structure with shadowing (when larger than 3 mm)

Note any free fluid accumulation in Morrison's pouch or the spleno-renal recess

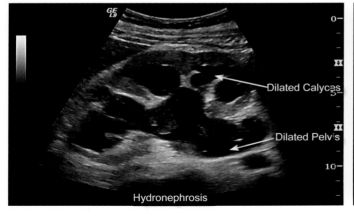

Hydronephrosis

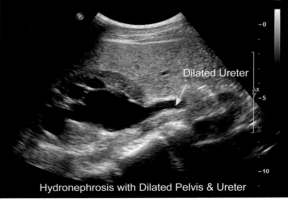

Hydronephrosis with Dilated Pelvis & Ureter

Work Sheet

Patient Name: _____
MRN: _____
Date: _____
Time: _____
History: _____
Vitals: HR   PB   RR   TEMP
US Performer: _____

FAST Exam

Positive Intraperitoneal Fluid:	☐Y	☐N
Estimated Volume/Measured # cm:		
Perihepatic:	☐Y	☐N
Perisplenic:	☐Y	☐N
Pelvic:	☐Y	☐N
Positive Subxiphoid view:	☐Y	☐N
Positive FAST ☐ Negative FAST ☐		

Extended FAST (E-FAST) Exam
Lung Exam

Right Pleural Effusion:	☐Y	☐N
Left Pleural Effusion:	☐Y	☐N
Pneumothorax	☐Y	☐N
Lung Sliding (right}	☐Y	☐N
Lung Sliding (left)	☐Y	☐N

IVC Diameter _____ cm

Respiratory change:	☐Y	☐N _____ % change
Collapse > 50%:	☐Y	☐N

GB & CBD

Gallstones:	☐Y	☐N
Sonographic Murphy's Sign:	☐Y	☐N
Pericholecystic Fluid:	☐Y	☐N
GB Wall thickness _____ cm		
Common Bile Duct Size _____ cm		

Pancreas

Parenchymal Abnormality:	☐Y	☐N
Head ☐ Uncinate Process ☐ Body ☐ Tail ☐		
Peripancreatic Fluid:	☐Y	☐N
Pseudocyst:	☐Y	☐N

Renal

Kidney Measurement (Long Axis):	☐Y	☐N
Hydronephrosis:	☐Y	☐N
Renal Stones:	Rt ☐ Lt ☐ Size _____	
Ureter Obstruction:	☐Y	☐N

Impression and comments:

Evaluation of The Aorta

Victor Coba M.D.

Contents

Indications

Suspicion of abdominal aortic aneurysm (AAA) with

- Abdominal pain

- Age >50

- Pulsatile mass

- Hypotension

- Back pain / Flank pain

Aorta

Patient Position

Supine

Transducer Type and Placement

Curvilinear or Phase Array

A6 /see abdominal chapter for transducer placement positions

- **Long Axis**
  - Transducer marker cephalad
- **Short Axis**
  - Transducer marker toward the patient's right

Depth 15-20 cm

Structures to be identified

Aorta
IVC
Spine
Celiac trunk
SMA
Renal arteries
Iliac arteries
Liver
Pancreas

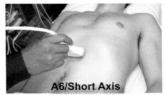

A6/Short Axis

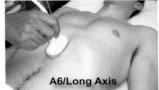

A6/Long Axis

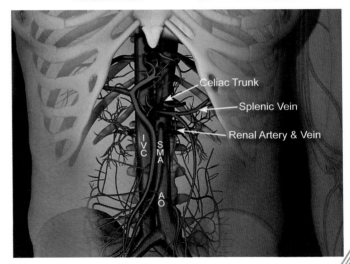

Celiac Trunk

Splenic Vein

Renal Artery & Vein

IVC   SMA   AO

Aorta

Sonographic Findings

The Aorta has a thicker wall compared to the IVC and is more circular and pulsatile

CF help identify the aorta and IVC

Normal maximal diameter is < 2 cm using anterior-posterior (AP) measurement **(outer wall to outer wall)**

- The diameter usually tapers down from proximal to distal

- Measure the diameter in long and short axis in all segments

Dilated aorta is >2 cm

Aneurysm is > 3 cm

Note the presence of a **flap** if aortic dissection is suspected

US is not sensitive in the diagnosis of rupture

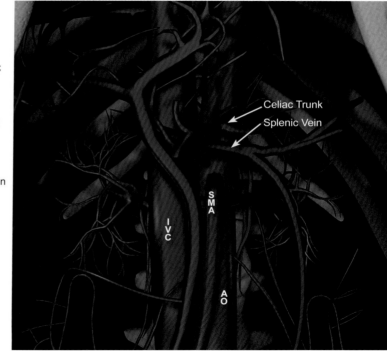

Celiac Trunk
Splenic Vein
S M A
I V C
A O

Aorta

Sonographic Findings (cont.)/Aortic sweep

Proximal segment

Just below the Xiphoid

Contains the **celiac trunk** and the superior mesenteric artery **(SMA)**

long axis

- The transducer marker cephalad
- Note the celiac trunk and the SMA

Aneurysms in this segment are not common

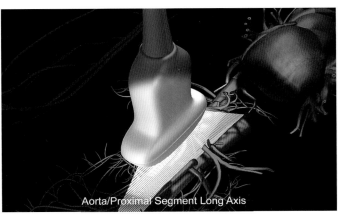

Aorta/Proximal Segment Long Axis

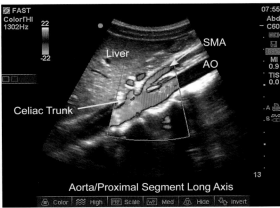

Aorta/Proximal Segment Long Axis

Aorta

Sonographic findings (cont.)/Aortic sweep

Proximal segment

Short Axis

- Rotating the transducer 90° CCW
- Note the celiac trunk
- Sliding the transducer downward will show the origin of the SMA (in transverse view)
- Measure the maximal A-P diameter, superior to the origin of the SMA

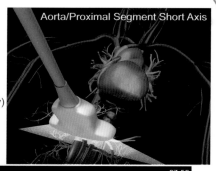

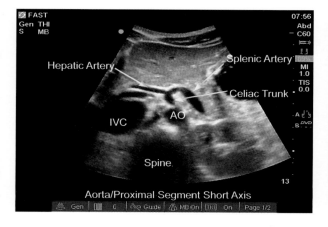

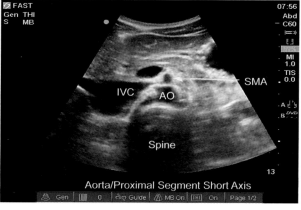

Aorta

Sonographic findings (cont.)/Aortic sweep

Middle segment

- Distal to the SMA origin
- Transducer pointing towards the spine with the marker towards the patient's right, slide transducer downward
- No branches recognized
- Measure the AP diameter in long and short axis
- The **renal arteries** originate very close to the origin of the SMA

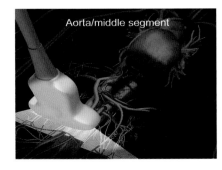

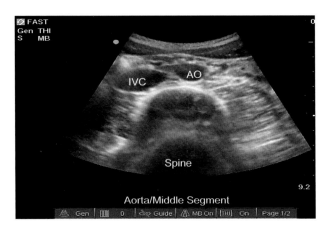

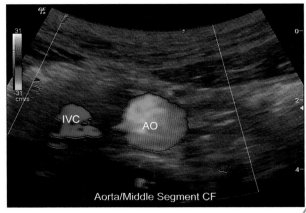

Aorta

Sonographic findings (cont.)/Aortic sweep

Distal Segment

- Aorta bifurcating into the iliac arteries, at or just below the umbilicus

- Continue same orientation (marker pointing towards patient's right), sliding the transducer downward

- More than **90%** of AAAs are infrarenal in the distal aorta.

- Measure the **largest A-P** diameter in long and short axis

- Bowel loops and gas may interfere with the view, and can be displaced by gentle pressure

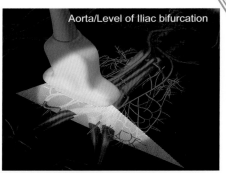

Aorta/Level of Iliac bifurcation

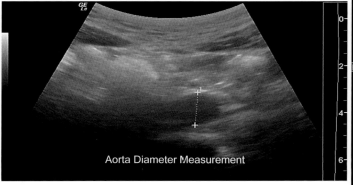

Aorta Diameter Measurement

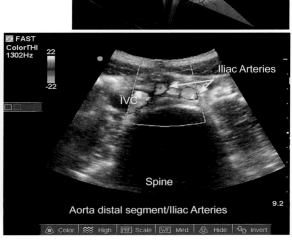

FAST
ColorTHI
1302Hz
22
-22

IVC

Iliac Arteries

Spine

Aorta distal segment/Iliac Arteries

9.2

Color | High | PRF Scale | WF Med | Hide | Invert

Evaluation of Aorta

Left Parasternal long Axis View

Transducer position

Start location: **C1**

Sonographic Findings

Examine the aortic valve, root, ascending aorta and part of the descending aorta

Normal aortic root diameter measurement is < 3.4 cm

Examine for the presence of any dissection or moving flap

Use CF to help visualize the flow and false lumen

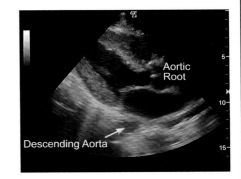

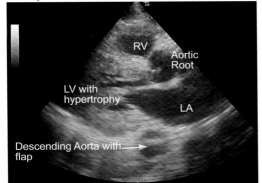

Parasternal long axis view/ Descending Aortic Dissection

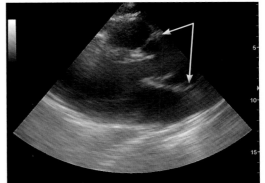

Parasternal Long Axis View/Dilated Aortic Root

Evaluation of the Aorta

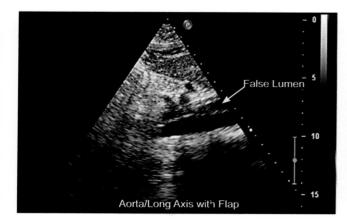

Aorta/Long Axis with Flap

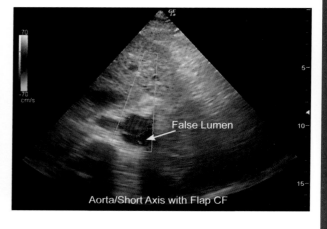

Aorta/Short Axis with Flap CF

Worksheet

Patient Name: _____
MRN: _____
Date: _____
Ultrasound Performer: _____

History
AP measurements (short axis)

Proximal _____ cm
Mid _____ cm
Distal _____ cm

AP measurements (long axis)

Proximal _____ cm
Mid _____ cm
Distal _____ cm

Abdominal Aortic Aneurysm   ☐ Y   ☐ N

Infrarenal ☐   Suprarenal ☐   Thoracoabdominal ☐

Common Iliacs   Normal ☐   Aneurysm ☐

Free Intraperitoneal Fluid   ☐ Y   ☐ N

Impression and comments:

Vascular Access

Keith Killu M.D.

Advantages of Vascular US

Identify anatomical variations

Decrease procedure failure rate

Decrease procedure related complications

Decrease procedure time

Decrease the number of attempts

Patient comfort

Contents

Equipment/Patient Position

Equipment

The transducer used in most vascular access procedures is the **linear** type 7-13 MHz

- The higher frequency is for better resolution

Sterile sheath, gel and rubber bands

Needle guide adaptors to guide the approach if desired

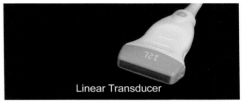

Linear Transducer

Patient Position

Position the patient in the optimal position depending on the location of the vessel accessed and the desired anatomical approach (e.g. Internal Jugular Vein access, place the patient in a Trendelenburg position)

The ultrasound machine placed where the operator can easily visualize the screen

Perform a scan of the vessel before starting the sterilization process to identify the largest diameter, relation to other vessels and the presence or absence of a thrombus

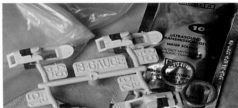

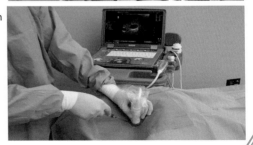

Pre-Procedure

Screen marker to the left

- Structures on the left of the screen are on the right side of the patient
- Depth is usually 3-4 cm

Orient yourself

- Obtain transverse and longitudinal views

By placing the vessel in the **center** of the screen, the transducer will be directly above it

Note the **depth of the vessel** (The right side of the screen will display the depth in centimeters)

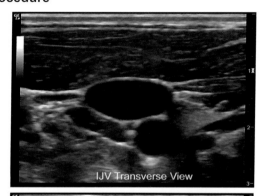

IJV Transverse View

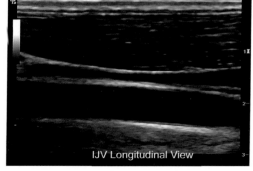

IJV Longitudinal View

Pre-Procedure

Using color flow (CF), orientation

When applying Color Flow, the top of the box on the left of the screen will indicate the color of the flow towards the transducer, and the bottom of the box indicates the color of the flow away from the transducer. In this example the Flow towards the transducer is red, and the flow away from the transducer is blue

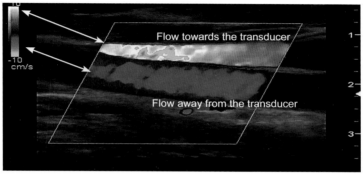

Dynamic vs Static Procedure

Dynamic (real time)

Sonographic localization and image guided cannulation
  - More precise
  - More difficult to maintain sterility
  - Need hand-eye coordination
  - One or two operators
  - The preferred method

Static (prescan, the procedure is done separately)

Ultrasonic localization of landmarks
  - Cannulation is separate
  - Easier to maintain sterility
  - Less technical demand
  - Less equipment needed

Sterile Kit/Needle Giude

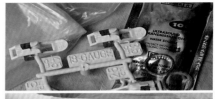

Sterile kit usually includes

- Sterile sheath
- Sterile gel
- Rubber bands
- Needle guides with different angle paths for different depths

Place the **gel** inside the sterile sheath

Place the sterile sheath on the transducer head and roll the sheath along the entire transducer cable

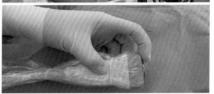

Place the **rubber bands**, one near the face and the other near the base of the transducer

Place sterile gel outside the sheath along the transducer head

Use a **Needle Guide** if desired

The needle guide is to be attached to the transducer head

The needle tip is placed through the guide

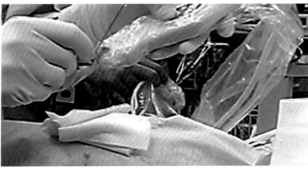

Advantages:

Predictable path, depth and angle of the needle

Less hand eye coordination needed

Disadvantages:

Angle is fixed

Deeper structures are hard to reach

Transducer Position & Orientation

The **Screen marker** is placed to the **left** of the screen. The Transducer marker pointing to the right side of the patient. Make sure the transducer marker side corresponds to the left side of the screen by touching the transducer footprint near the transducer marker

Always maintain universal sterile precautions

Transducer held in the non dominant hand and the needle in the dominant hand

Transducer should be perpendicular and in complete contact with the skin

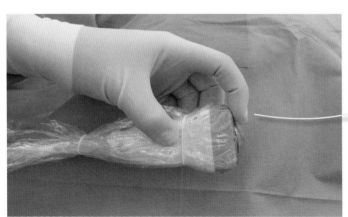
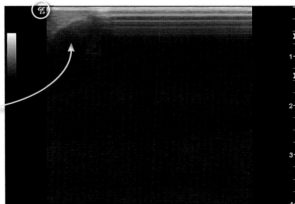

Procedure/Differentiate the Artery from the Vein

The **vein** is usually

- Oval in shape, thin walled
- Compressible with gentle pressure
- Non pulsatile
- Valsalva maneuver can increase the neck vein size

The **artery** is usually

- Circular in shape, thicker wall
- Non compressible, pulsatile

Use **CF** to demonstrate blood flow direction and pulsation

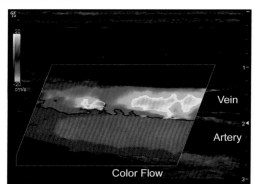

Vein

Artery

Color Flow

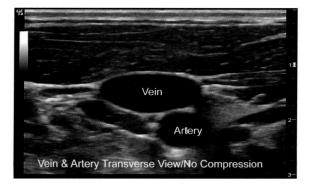

Vein & Artery Transverse View/No Compression

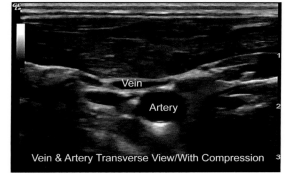

Vein & Artery Transverse View/With Compression

Differentiate the artery from the Vein
Pulse Wave Doppler (PW)

Pulse Wave (PW) Doppler generates audible signals and wave forms to help differentiate an artery from a vein

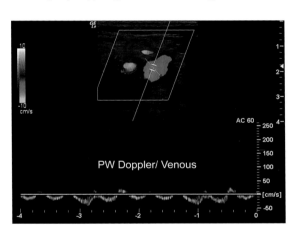

PW Doppler/ Venous

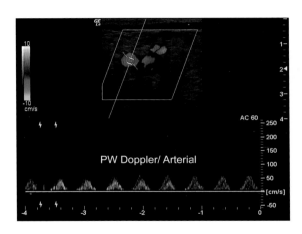

PW Doppler/ Arterial

Differentiate blood Vessels from Nerves

Nerves are generally more difficult to identify

Use blood vessels and bony landmarks to identify adjacent neural structures

Usually **oval or round** in shape, non compressible and has no color flow

More echogenic than blood vessels

Echogenicity depends on the transcucer angle and the nerve size (larger nerves are more echogenic)

Note the hypo-echoic **Fascicles** that look like grapes forming the nerve bundle surrounded by hyper-echoic connective tissue sheath

Median nerve near the wrist or in the forearm is a good start and reference for learning

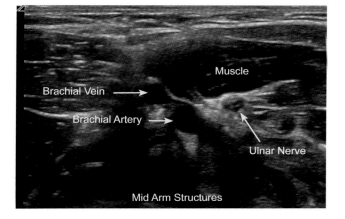

Muscle

Brachial Vein ⟶

Brachial Artery ⟶

Ulnar Nerve

Mid Arm Structures

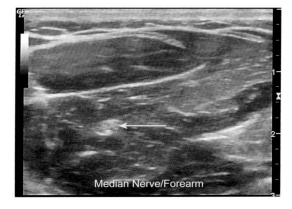

Median Nerve/Forearm

Procedure/Localizing the Vessel

Place the transducer perpendicular to the skin

To prevent transducer sliding, place part of the hand holding the transducer on the skin

View the vessel in a **long and short axis view**

Note the **depth** of the vessel

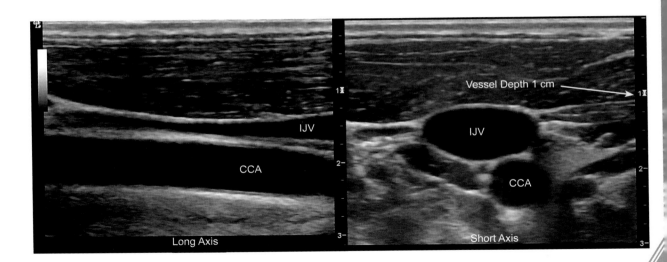

Procedure/Long vs. Short Axis

Long Axis view

- Provides a better needle slope positioning and can monitor the needle throughout the procedure
- Tip of the needle is easier to localize
- More difficult for hand eye coordination

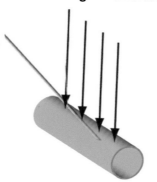

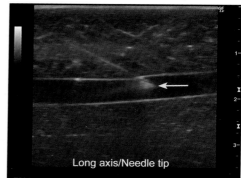

Long axis/Needle tip

Short Axis view

- Preferred for dynamic line placement
- Allows for a better lateral positioning of the needle
- Tip of the needle is harder to localize
- Easier hand eye coordination

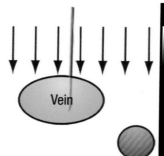

Vein

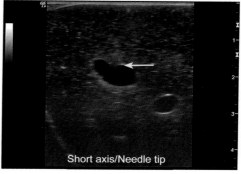

Short axis/Needle tip

Procedure/Insertion method

Apply **local anesthetic**

Place the needle 1-2 cm behind the transducer with the **bevel facing upwards**

Angle the needle at about 45°-60° from the skin

Sometimes the angle is steeper when trying to avoid another structure

Perform a mock poke and notice the **ring down** artifact to locate the needle

Anatomical landmark approach is not always applied since you are in full view of the vessel

Needle should be moved in short slow controlled fashion

Locate the tip of the needle (which may appear as an echogenic dot)

Place the bevel towards the transducer beam which will produce more echo return and better visualization of the needle tip

If the needle can't be visualized, readjust the transducer, gently wiggle the needle or change its angle

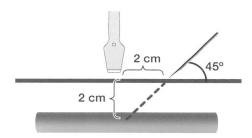

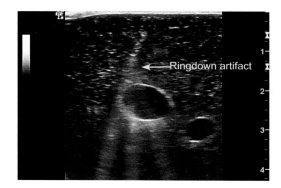

Internal Jugular Vein (IJV)

Patient Position

Place the patient in a supine position for pre procedure scanning, then in a trendelenburg position for the procedure

Transducer Type & Placement

Linear Transducer 7-13 MHz

Short Axis

- Transducer marker pointing towards the patient's **left** (One of the few instances where the marker points towards the patient's left. This is done because the position of the operator **is at the head of the bed**

Long Axis

- Transducer marker pointing cephalad

Screen marker to the left of the screen

Depth 2-4 cm

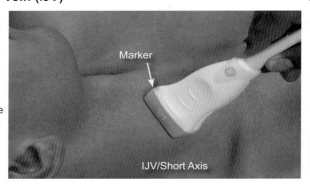

IJV/Short Axis

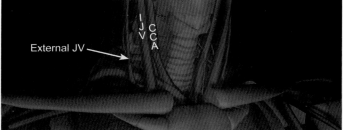

External JV

I J V
C C A

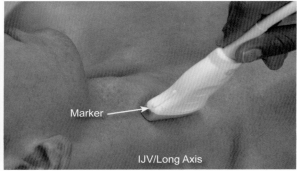

Marker

IJV/Long Axis

IJV/Long and Short Axis

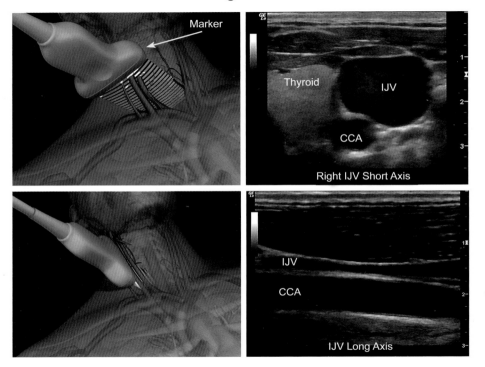

Marker

Thyroid
IJV
CCA

Right IJV Short Axis

IJV
CCA

IJV Long Axis

IJV/CF, PW

Apply **CF** to help differentiate the artery from the vein

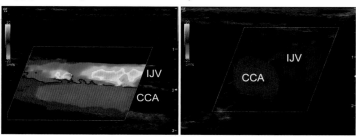

Continue the line placement with the standard Seldinger technique

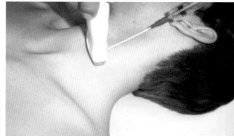

Pulse wave (PW) Doppler generates audible signals and waveforms to help differentiate the artery from the vein

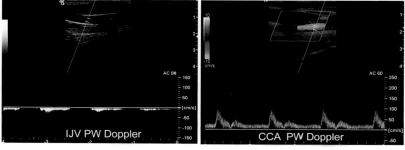

IJV/Catheter Position

Post procedure, it is possible sometimes to locate the catheter or it's tip in the superior vena cava (SVC)

- **Transducer Placement**

   Place the transducer between the two heads or lateral to the sternocleidomastoid muscle with the ultrasound beam directed towards the back of the sternum.

Depth usually about **8 cm**

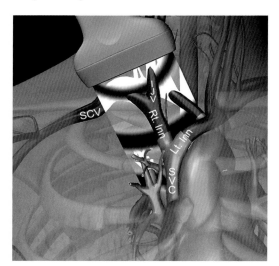

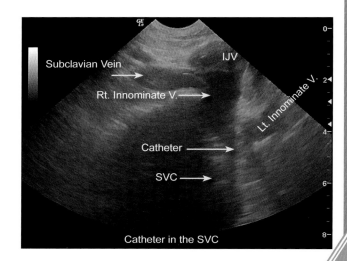

Catheter in the SVC

IJV/Post procedure

Check for **pneumothorax** post procedure

- Apply the transducer to the anterior chest wall in the 2nd-8th intercostal spaces mid clavicular line **(L1,L2),** and 4th-10th spaces **(L3)** anterior and mid axillary lines

  - **"Lung Sliding" Sign/B-Mode**

    - Two echogenic pleural lines sliding with respiration

  - **Seashore Sign/M-Mode**

- Presence of lung sliding and the seashore sign usually **rules out** the presence of pneumothorax

- Refer to the lung chapter for more details

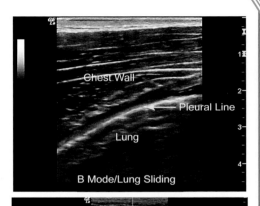

Chest Wall
Pleural Line
Lung
B Mode/Lung Sliding

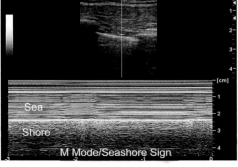

Sea
Shore
M Mode/Seashore Sign

Subclavian vein

Patient Position

Place the patient in a supine position for pre procedure scanning, then in a trendelenburg position for the procedure

Transducer Type & Position

Linear Transducer 7-13 MHz

Place the transducer perpendicular to the skin, at the lateral aspect of the clavicle outside the thoracic cage

Short Axis View

- Transducer marker pointing cephalad

Long axis View

- Transducer marker towards the patient's right

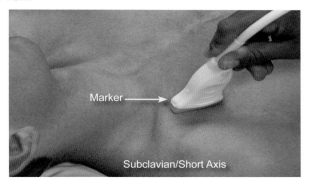

Subclavian/Short Axis

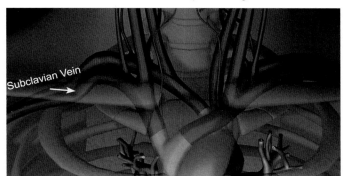

Subclavian Vein

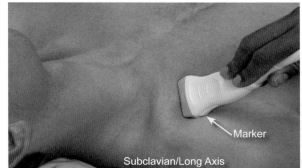

Subclavian/Long Axis

Subclavian vein

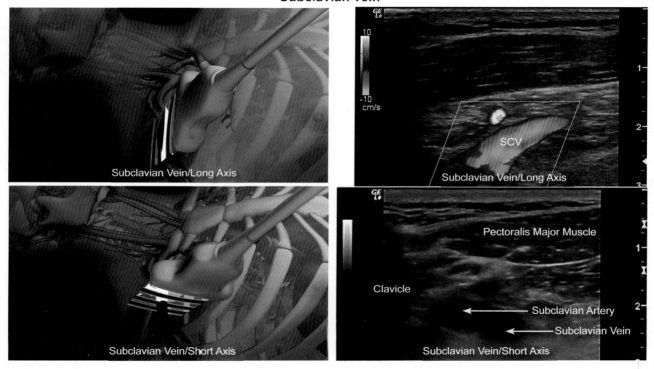

Subclavian Vein/Long Axis

Subclavian Vein/Long Axis

SCV

Subclavian Vein/Short Axis

Pectoralis Major Muscle

Clavicle

Subclavian Artery

Subclavian Vein

Subclavian Vein/Short Axis

Subclavian vein

Procedure

The subclavian vein is somewhat difficult to scan

Better to prescan and locate the vessel, then do the procedure separately

Apply **CF, PW** Doppler and compression to help differentiate the artery from the vein

Obtain a long and a short axis views

Once the vessel is identified, Continue line placement with the standard Seldinger technique

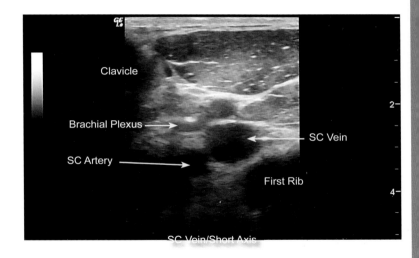

Subclavian vein /Supraclavicular approach

Patient Position
Place the patient in a supine position for scanning, then in a Trendelenburg position with preferably a small towel between the shoulder blades for the procedure

Transducer Type & Placement
Linear Transducer
Place the transducer perpendicular to the skin, at the medial aspect of the clavicle outside the thoracic cage

Short Axis View
• Transducer marker pointing cephalad

Long Axis View
• Transducer marker towards the patient's right

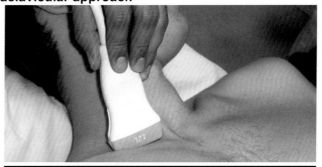

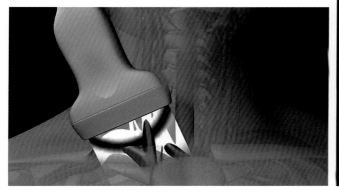

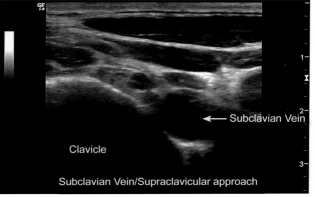

← Subclavian Vein

Clavicle

Subclavian Vein/Supraclavicular approach

Femoral Vein & Artery

Patient Position

Place the patient in supine position

Transducer Type & Placement

Linear transducer

Transducer placed just inferior to the inguinal ligament and the marker towards the patient's right

Screen marker to the left

Depth 4-6 cm depending on the body habitus

Short Axis

- Transducer marker towards the patient's right

Long Axis

- Transducer marker cephalad

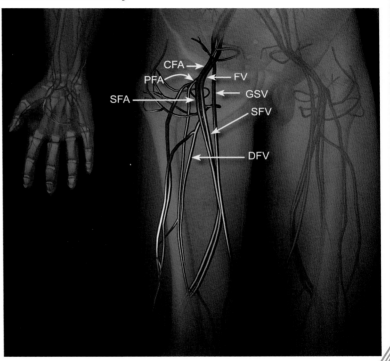

Femoral Vein & Artery

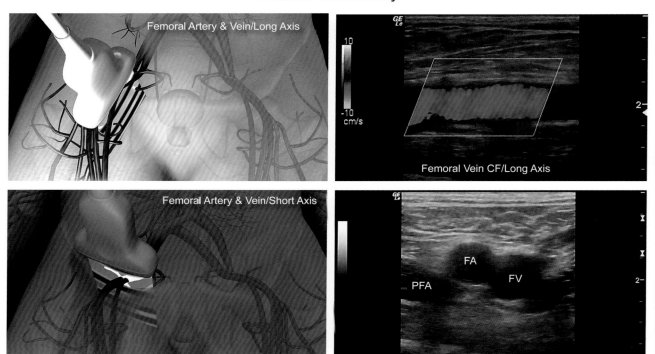

Femoral Artery & Vein/Long Axis

Femoral Vein CF/Long Axis

Femoral Artery & Vein/Short Axis

PFA FA FV

Femoral Vein & Artery

Procedure

Vein is medial to the artery

Obtain a long and short axis view

Using CF, PW Doppler and compression can help differentiate between the artery and the vein

Once the vessel is identified, Continue line placement following the standard Seldinger technique

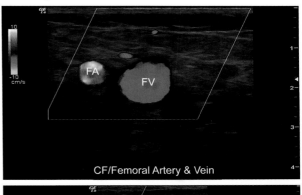

CF/Femoral Artery & Vein

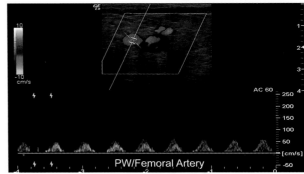

PW/Femoral Artery

Radial Artery

Patient Position

Place the forearm on a solid surface with the wrist slightly extended

Transducer Type & Placement

Linear transducer

Transducer marker towards the patient's right

Depth 2-3 cm

Prescan and identify the radial artery

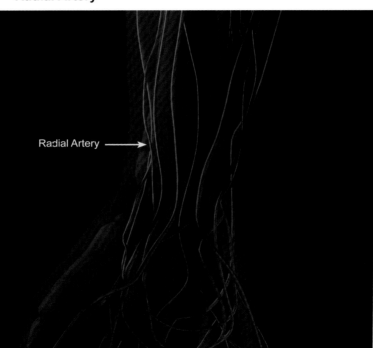

Radial Artery →

Radial Artery

Obtain short and long axis for better orientation specially with narrow vessels

Once the vessel is identified, continue line placement following the standard technique

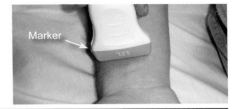

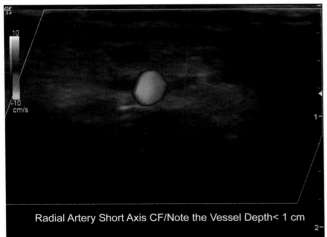

Radial Artery Short Axis CF/Note the Vessel Depth< 1 cm

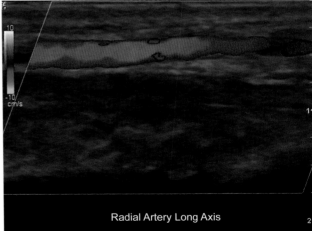

Radial Artery Long Axis

Axillary Artery

Patient Position

Place the patient in supine position

Head turned 30° to the opposite side

Arm abducted 90° and externally rotated with the elbow flexed

Transducer Type & Placement

Linear transducer

Place the transducer close to the axilla to access the **2nd or 3rd part** of the axillary artery.

Transducer marker pointing upward

Depth 2-3 cm

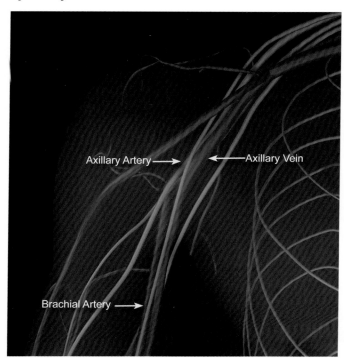

Axillary Artery

Procedure

Access will mostly be in the 2nd & 3rd parts of the axillary artery

Note the pulsating axillary artery, the compressible axillary vein, nerve bundle with the ulnar nerve (inferior & medial) and median nerve (superior & lateral)

Apply adequate local anesthesia

Place the needle behind the transducer, puncture the skin and follow the needle's path

Continue the procedure following the standard technique

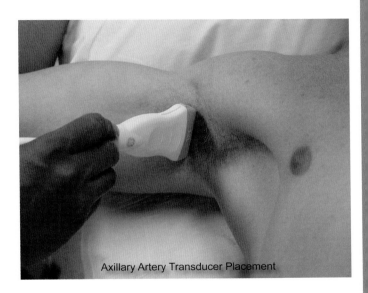

Axillary Artery Transducer Placement

Axillary Artery

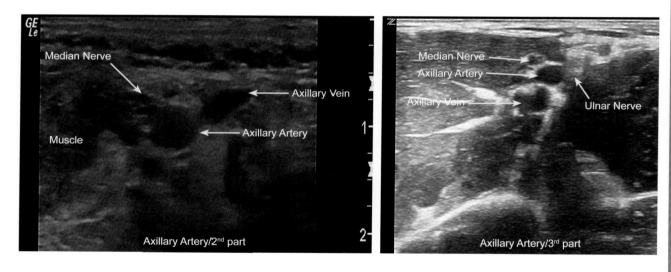

Peripherally Inserted Central Catheter (PICC)

Patient Position

Supine

The arm should be abducted 90° and externally rotated with the elbow flexed

Place a tourniquet as close to the axilla as possible

Transducer Type & Placement

Linear transducer

Transducer placed in the short axis of the arm with the marker pointing upwards

Depth 2-3 cm

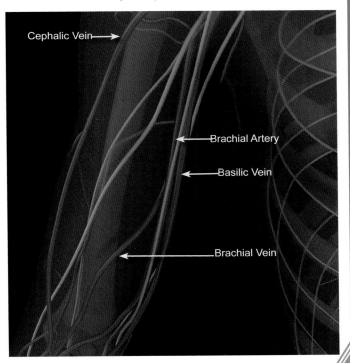

Cephalic Vein

Brachial Artery

Basilic Vein

Brachial Vein

PICC

Procedure

Map the entire arm to find the best position for insertion

- Basilic (first choice)
- Cephalic vein
- Deep brachial veins
- Identify the Arteries

Measure the distance from the insertion site to the acromion process then add 20 cm (this will represent the length of the catheter to be inserted)

Continue line placement following the standard technique

Verify the catheter position in the SVC by fluoroscopy, CXR or ultrasound

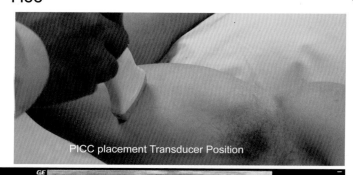

PICC placement Transducer Position

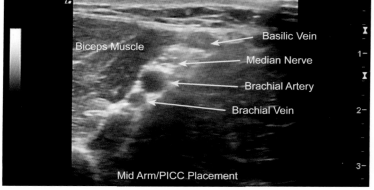

Biceps Muscle
Basilic Vein
Median Nerve
Brachial Artery
Brachial Vein

Mid Arm/PICC Placement

Peripheral Veins

Peripheral vein access using a cannula can be made easy by using ultrasound to locate the vessel

Transducer Type & Placement

Linear transducer

Placed directly over the vein site with the marker towards the patient's right

Depth 1-2 cm

Can perform the procedure in the dynamic or static method

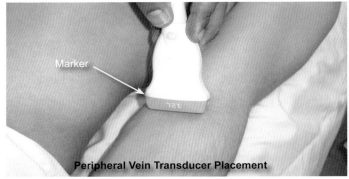

Peripheral Vein Transducer Placement

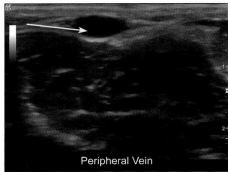

Peripheral Vein

Peripheral Veins

Most veins can be accessed using ultrasound guidance

Locating the vein and determining its depth will help avoid multiple attempts

Using **CF** and **PW Doppler** can help differentiate an artery from a vein

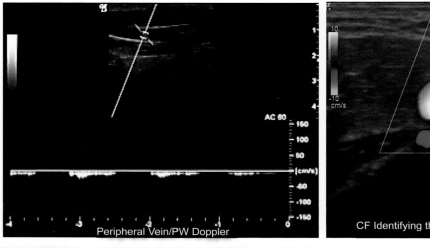

Peripheral Vein/PW Doppler

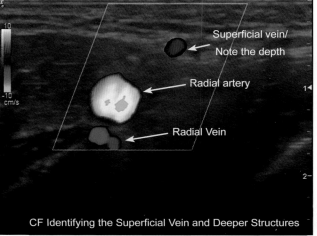

Superficial vein/ Note the depth

Radial artery

Radial Vein

CF Identifying the Superficial Vein and Deeper Structures

Lung Exam

Scott Dulchavsky, MD, PhD
Keith Killu, MD

Contents

Indications

To evaluate patients with respiratory compromise or failure

- Pulmonary edema, ARDS, alveolar interstitial disease
- Pleural effusion
- Pneumothorax
- Consolidation
- Diaphragmatic dysfunction

Part of the Extended-FAST exam

Procedure guidance

Evaluation of the patient's fluid status

Lung zones & Transducer types

Lung Examination Zones

Always examine both lungs. The transducer should be perpendicular to the chest wall

Lung Zone 1/L1

2nd, 3rd, 4th intercostal spaces, anterior chest wall

Lung Zone 2/L2

5th-8th intercostal spaces, anterior chest wall

Lung Zone 3/L3

4th-10th intercostal spaces, between the anterior & posterior axillary lines

Lung Zone 4/L4

Posterior chest wall. Mainly for procedure guidance in pleurocentesis

Different references will give different lung zones. We found these to be the easiest, and most practical to cover most of the clinical applications in the ICU

Patient Position

Supine

Transducer type

Curvilinear, Microconvex or Phased Array
- For deeper structures

Linear
- For superficial structures (pleura)

Ultrasound screen marker to the Left of the screen, and the depth should be about 10-15 cm

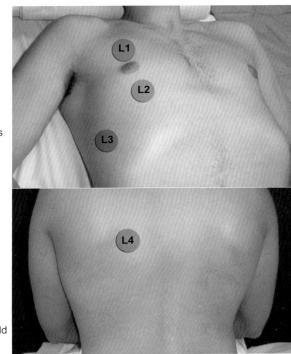

Transducer placement

Transducer Placement

Long axis

Place the transducer footprint perpendicular to the chest wall with the marker pointing cephalad

Short axis

Turn the transducer 90° CCW

Structures to be identified

Chest Wall

Pleura

Lung parenchyma

Diaphragm

Liver & Spleen

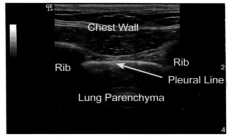

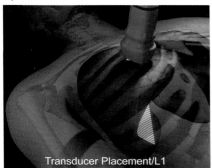

Transducer Placement/L1

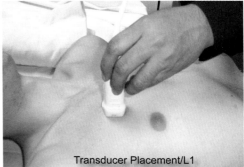

Transducer Placement/L1

Transducer placement

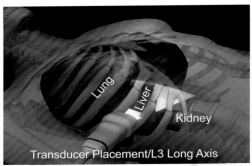

Transducer Placement/L3 Long Axis

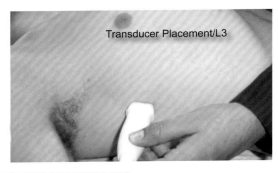

Transducer Placement/L3

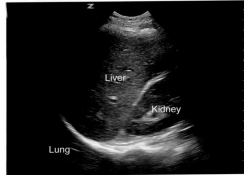

Lung Signs

Sonographic Findings/Lung Signs

Bat Sign/Normal

- Transducer at **L1**, with the marker Cephalad
- The sign is formed by the shadows of two ribs and the pleural line (looks like a bat flying towards you)
- Try to obtain this image initially, to avoid artifacts

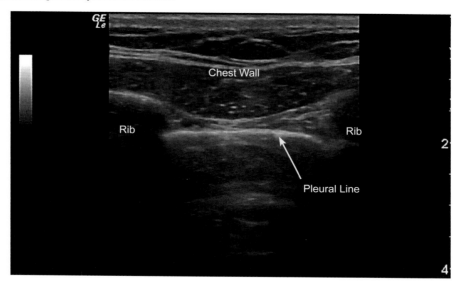

Lung Signs

Sonographic Findings/Lung Signs (cont.)

Lung Sliding/Normal

Pleural line is found below the chest wall

Movement of pleura with breathing will generate the "lung sliding" sign

- Represents the sliding of the visceral pleura against the parietal pleura
- Using Color Flow (CF) can help identify the pleural line and its movement
- Best seen near the lung bases
- Can be **absent** in pneumothorax, atelectasis, pleurodesis, parietal emphysema or any cause that interrupts the normal pleural movement

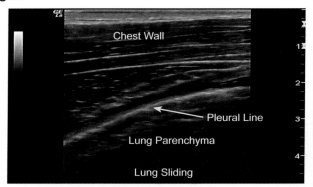

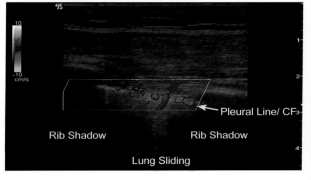

Lung Signs

Sonographic Findings/Lung Signs

Lung Sliding (cont.)

- Lung sliding can sometimes be better evaluated with the **M Mode** generating the **"Sea Shore"** sign
- The presence of lung sliding and the sea shore sign, mostly rules out pneumothorax

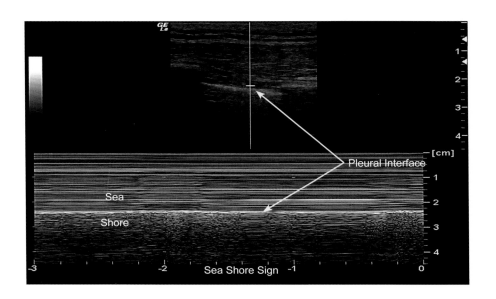

Lungs Signs

Sonographic Findings/Lung Signs (cont.)

A Lines/Normal

Can be part of the normal lung signs

Represents normal artifact repetition(s) of the pleural line

Intervals between the A lines are equal to the distance between the skin and the original pleural line

When present without lung sliding, it may indicate the presence of pneumothorax

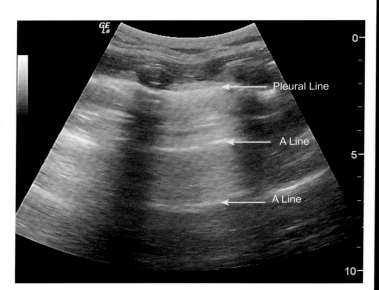

Lung Signs

Sonographic Findings/Lung Signs (cont.)

Comet Tail Artifact/B Lines

- Vertical lines, extending from the pleural line to the edge of the screen without fading

- Synchronized with lung sliding

- When present they will usually overshadow the A lines

- Represents thickening interlobular septa and extravascular lung water as in alveolar interstitial disease (pulmonary edema, ARDS...)

- Their presence mostly rules out pneumothorax

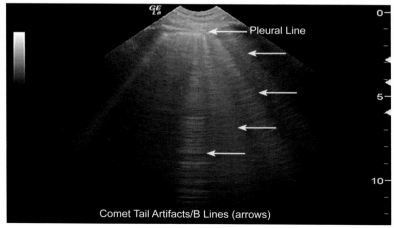

Comet Tail Artifacts/B Lines (arrows)

Lung Signs

Sonographic Findings/Lung Signs (cont.)

Z Lines

- Represents artifacts
- Originates from the pleural line, fades after few centimeters
- Do not extend to the edge of the screen
- Do not overshadow the A lines

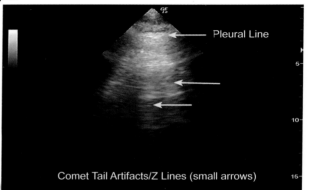

Comet Tail Artifacts/Z Lines (small arrows)

Lung and Pleural Profiles Summary

A Profile = designate anterior predominant A lines associated with lung sliding e.g., COPD, asthma, + DVT = PE

A' Profile = A profile with abolished lung sliding e.g., pneumothorax

B Profile = Bilateral anterior B lines with lung sliding, e.g., pulmonary edema

B' Profile = B profile with no lung sliding e.g., pneumonia. atelectasis

A/B Profile = B lines on one side, A lines on the other e.g., pneumonia

C Profile = anterior alveolar consolidation e.g., pneumonia, atelectasis

Pleural Effusion

Patient Position
Supine

Pulmonary regions
Lung Zones **L3, L4**

Transducer Type & Placement
Phased Array or Curvilinear

The footprint is perpendicular to the skin with the marker pointing cephalad

Start at the lower edge of zone **L3** and slide the transducer cephalad to detect the interface between the diaphragm and pleural space

Structures to be identified
Chest Wall

Diaphragm

Lung

Pleural effusion

Liver or spleen

Sonographic Findings
Anechoic space separating the parietal and visceral pleura

Note the lung movement with respiration **(Jelly Fish Sign)**

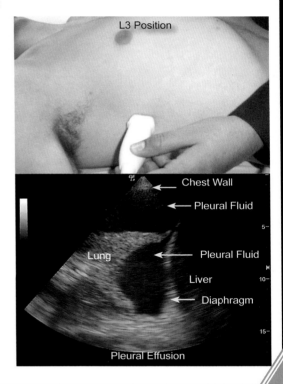

L3 Position

Chest Wall

Pleural Fluid

Lung

Pleural Fluid

Liver

Diaphragm

Pleural Effusion

Pleural Effusion

Sonographic Findings (cont.)

Note the **Quad sign** on 2D, the pleural effusion is delineated by the pleural line (upper border), lung line (lower border) and the two rib shadows

Note the Sinusoid sign on **M Mode**

- Represents **movement of the floating lung** towards the chest wall with respiration

- Specific for pleural effusion

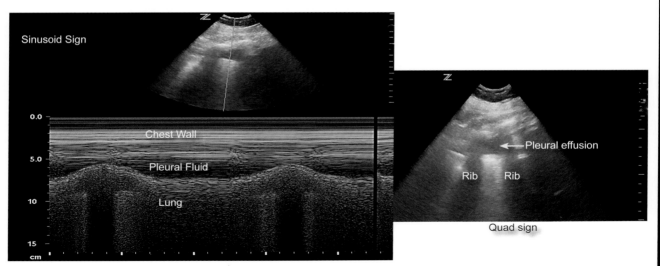

Quad sign

Pleural Effusion

Sonographic Findings (cont.)

Fluid Nature
Transudate
- Completely anechoic

Exudate
- Can be anechoic
- Usually echoic with particles

Purulent Pleurisy
- Echoic
- Presence of septations
- Not uncommonly a honey comb pattern

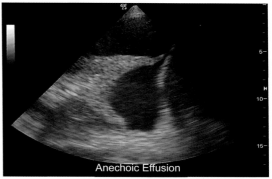
Anechoic Effusion

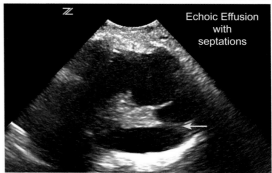
Echoic Effusion with septations

Pleural Effusion

Sonographic Findings (cont.)

Fluid Volume

Measure the fluid depth at the lung base or the level of the 5th intercostal space

Measurement starts 3 cm from the inferior pole of the lung to the chest wall

> 5 cm fluid thickness indicate pleural effusion **> 500 ml**

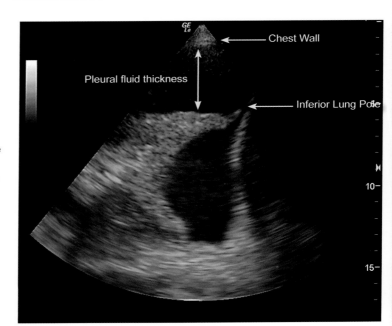

Chest Wall

Pleural fluid thickness

Inferior Lung Pole

Pneumothorax

In a critically ill supine patient, air tends to accumulate in the anterior portion of the thorax

The diagnosis is made by detecting the absence of the lung tissue movement beneath the pleural line

Patient Position

Supine

Transducer

Linear 7-13 MHz, for pleural interface

Phased Array 2.5-5 MHz or
Curvilinear 2-5 MHz

Transducer Placement

Perpendicular to the skin in Zones **L1, L2 & L3**

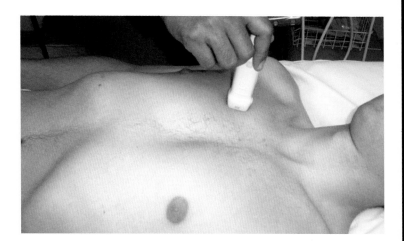

Pneumothorax

Structures to be identified

Pleura, Lung and Ribs

Sonographic Findings

Lung Sliding is absent . 100% sensitivity

- No lung sliding on **B Mode**

- Seashore sign on **M Mode** is replaced by the **Stratosphere sign** (no sand, all sea)

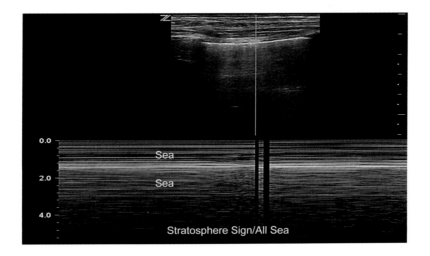

Pneumothorax

Sonographic Findings (cont.)
Lung Point

- A localized **transition** point from intrapleural air (pneumothorax artifact) to the interparanchymal air is **100% specific** for pneumothorax

- The transition from the seashore sign to the stratosphere sign on the **M Mode**

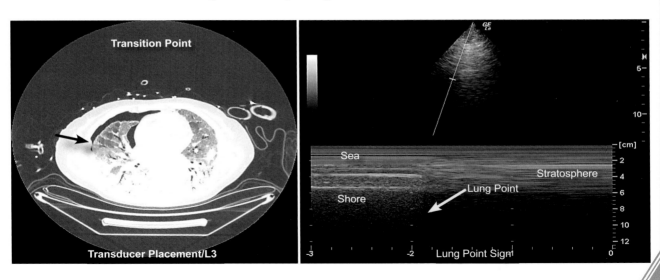

Acute Interstitial Syndrome

Indications

Pulmonary edema

ARDS

Pneumonia/Interstitial disease

Patient Position

Supine

Transducer type & placement

Phased Array 2.5-5 MHz or
Curvilinear 2-5 MHz

Perpendicular to the skin in Zones **L1, L2 & L3**

Sonographic Findings

B Lines

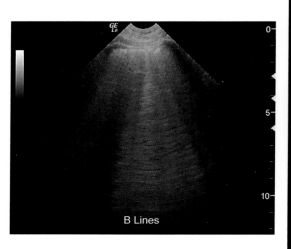

B Lines

- Vertical lines extending from the pleural line **to the edge of the screen** without fading, separated by an average distance of 7 mm or less

- To calculate the **Comet Tail Score**, count the number of the comet tails (B Lines) in lung zones **L1, L2, L3** bilaterally

   The higher the number, the more severe is the interstitial process

- Has a 93% sensitivity and specificity in patients with pulmonary edema

- Disappears after treatment of the underlying disorder

- Absent in patients with COPD

Acute Interstitial Syndrome

Sonographic Findings
ARDS/Pneumonia

- The lung tissue will resemble the hepatic parenchyma
- B Lines may be present
- In the case of associated pneumonia, Alveolar Consolidations with **air bronchogram** and possible **Shred sign** may be seen
- In most ICU patients, the area involved will be **L3**

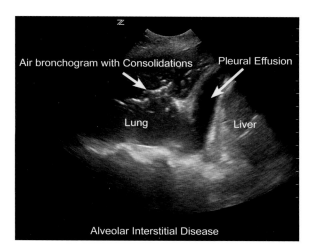

Alveolar Interstitial Disease

Acute Interstitial Syndrome

Sonographic findings (cont.)

Pneumonia

- Tissue like image arising from the pleural line
- Air bronchogram (hyperechoic artifacts) with **dynamic movement** with respiration
- **Shred signs** - Shredded tissue like pattern bordered by the pleural line, lung line and a deep irregular border
- **Focal B Profile**

Atelectasis

- Lung sliding will be absent
- **Lung pulse** (transmission of heartbeat to the pleural line)
- No dynamic movement of the air bronchogram

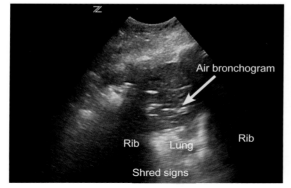

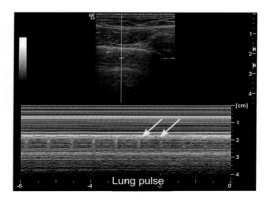

Diaphragm

Patient Position

Supine

Transducer

Phased Array 2.5-5 MHz

Transducer Placement

L3, marker pointing cephalad

The interface between the diaphragm and lung at about 5th to 8th intercostal space mid-posterior axillary line

Examine both sides

Structures to be identified

Lung

Diaphragm

Liver or spleen

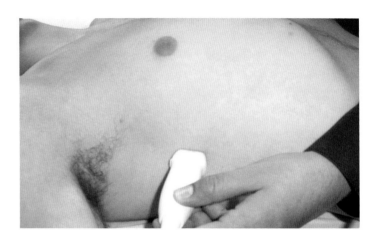

Diaphragm

Sonographic Findings

Inspiratory amplitude in normal spontaneously breathing patient s usually >10mm-20mm

Diaphragmatic Dysfunction

- Presence of pleural effusion does not usually affect this amplitude
- Amplitude < 5 mm is pathological
- There will be a diminished lung sliding and paradoxical movement
- M-Mode can be used to detect and measure the diaphragmatic movement

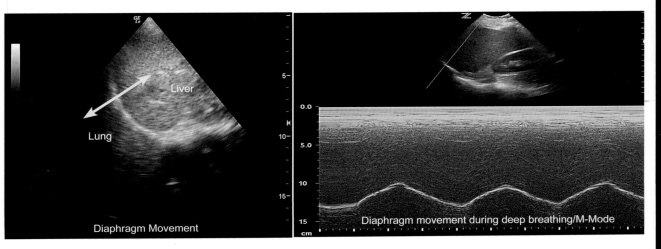

Diaphragm Movement

Diaphragm movement during deep breathing/M-Mode

Worksheet

Patient Name: _____

MRN: _____

Date: _____

History: _____

Vitals: _____

Lung, Pleural & Diaphragm limited exam

Normal	☐Y	☐N
Pleural Effusion	☐Y	☐N

☐ Rt. ☐Y ☐N Estimated Size....

☐ Lt. ☐Y ☐N Estimated Size....

Pneumothorax	☐Y	☐N	☐Rt ☐Lt
Lung Sliding	☐Y	☐N	
Stratosphere Sign	☐Y	☐N	
A lines	☐Y	☐N	
Lung Point	☐Y	☐N	

Acute Interstitial Pattern	☐Y	☐N
Right		
B Lines	☐Y	☐N
Consolidation	☐Y	☐N
Bronchograms	☐Y	☐N
Left		
B Lines	☐Y	☐N
Consolidation	☐Y	☐N
Bronchograms	☐Y	☐N
Diaphragm Dysfunction	☐Y	☐N

Impression, Comments and Recommendations:

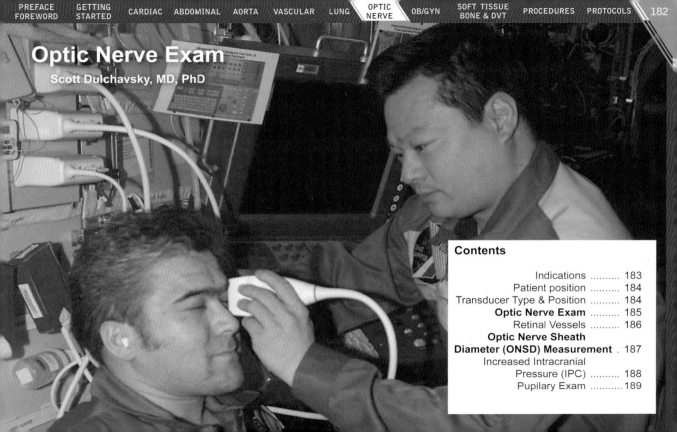

Optic Nerve Exam

Scott Dulchavsky, MD, PhD

Contents

Optic Nerve Exam

Indications

Evaluation of the optic disc

Evaluation of the Optic Nerve Sheath Diameter **(ONSD)**

Normal value < **5-5.7 mm**

Any cause that may lead to increased **ICP > 20** mmHg, will mostly lead to an increase in **ONSD > 5.7 mm**

- Traumatic Brain Injury (TBI)
- Intracranial bleeding
- Hydrocephalus
- Hypertensive emergency

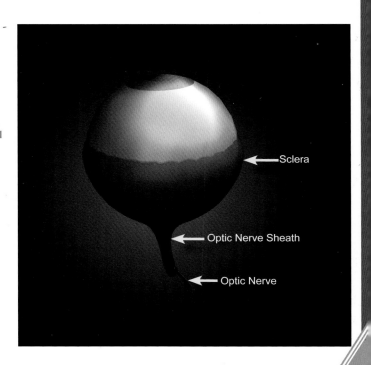

Sclera

Optic Nerve Sheath

Optic Nerve

Optic Nerve Exam

Patient Position

Supine

Transducer type and position

Linear 7-13 MHz

Apply the transducer directly to the closed eyelid

Sagittal Axis

- Transducer marker cephalad

Horizontal Axis

- Transducer marker towards the patient's right

Depth 3-4 cm

Use **ALARA** principle with the lowest amount of energy possible

- Mechanical index (MI) should be < 0.23 in opthalmic applications

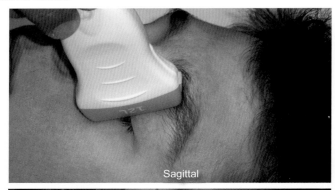

Sagittal

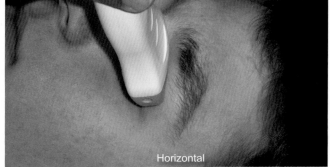

Horizontal

Optic Nerve Exam

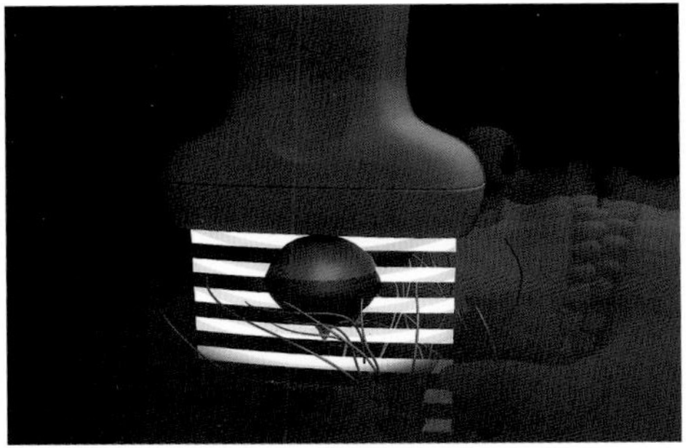

Structures to be identified

Cornea, Lens

Choroid & Retina

Optic disk

Optic Nerve

Optic Nerve Sheath **(ONS)**

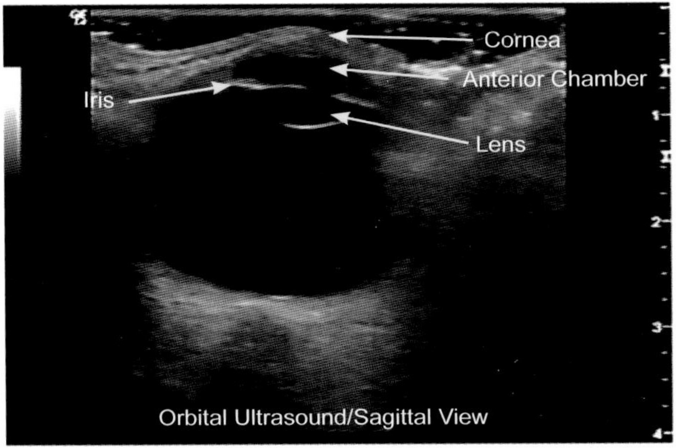
Cornea
Anterior Chamber
Iris
Lens
1
2
3
4

Orbital Ultrasound/Sagittal View

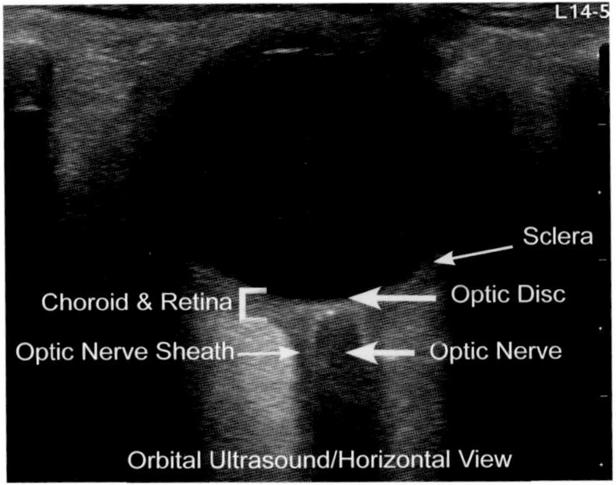
L14-5
Sclera
Choroid & Retina
Optic Disc
Optic Nerve Sheath
Optic Nerve

Orbital Ultrasound/Horizontal View

Optic Nerve Exam & Retinal vessels

Sonographic findings

Recommended to scan **both eyes**

Adjust the depth to fill the screen with the entire orbit

The **cornea** is seen as a thin layer parallel to the eyelid

The normal **lens** is anechoic

The normal eye appears as a circular **hypoechoic** structure

The **optic nerve** is visible posteriorly departing away from the globe and optic disc

Using Color Flow **(CF)** can help identify the Central retinal vessels

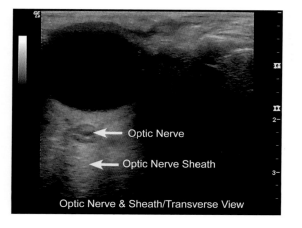

Optic Nerve & Sheath/Transverse View

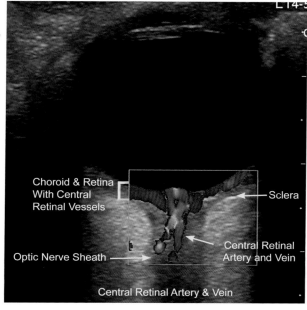

Central Retinal Artery & Vein

Optic Nerve Exam / ONSD Measurement

Sonographic findings (cont.)

ONSD measurement

Measurement of the ONSD should be done about 3mm posterior to the optic disc

Two measurements averaged in each of the Horizontal and Sagittal planes

A normal ONSD measures **< 5-5.7mm**

> 5.7mm may be indicative of **increased ICP** and a head CT is recommended

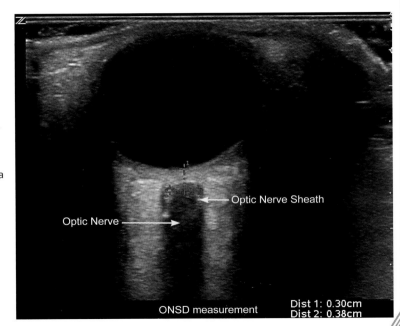

Optic Nerve Sheath

Optic Nerve

ONSD measurement

Dist 1: 0.30cm
Dist 2: 0.38cm

Optic Exam

Sonographic findings (cont.)

Other features of Traumatic Brain Injury **(TBI)** and **increased ICP** can be identified

- Swelling of the optic disk & Papilledema
- **Retinal detachment** can be identified
- **Vitreous hemorrhage** with opacities in the vitreous fluid can sometimes be seen

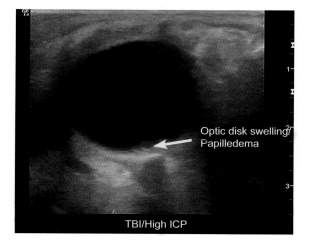

Optic disk swelling/ Papilledema

TBI/High ICP

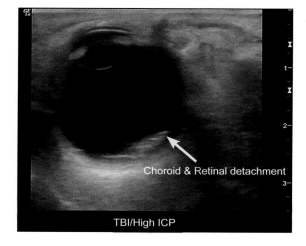

Choroid & Retinal detachment

TBI/High ICP

Optic Exam

Sonographic findings (cont.)

Examination of the **pupil** can be achieved by placing the transducer on the lower lid of the closed eye and angling superiorly (achieving a coronal plane with the globe and obtaining a view of the iris). This can help measure pupillary reflexes and accurately measure of pupil size by M mode

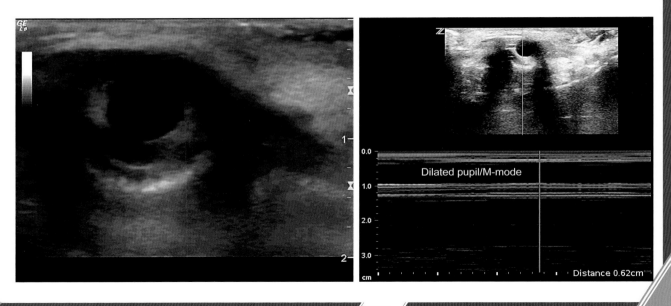

Dilated pupil/M-mode

Distance 0.62cm

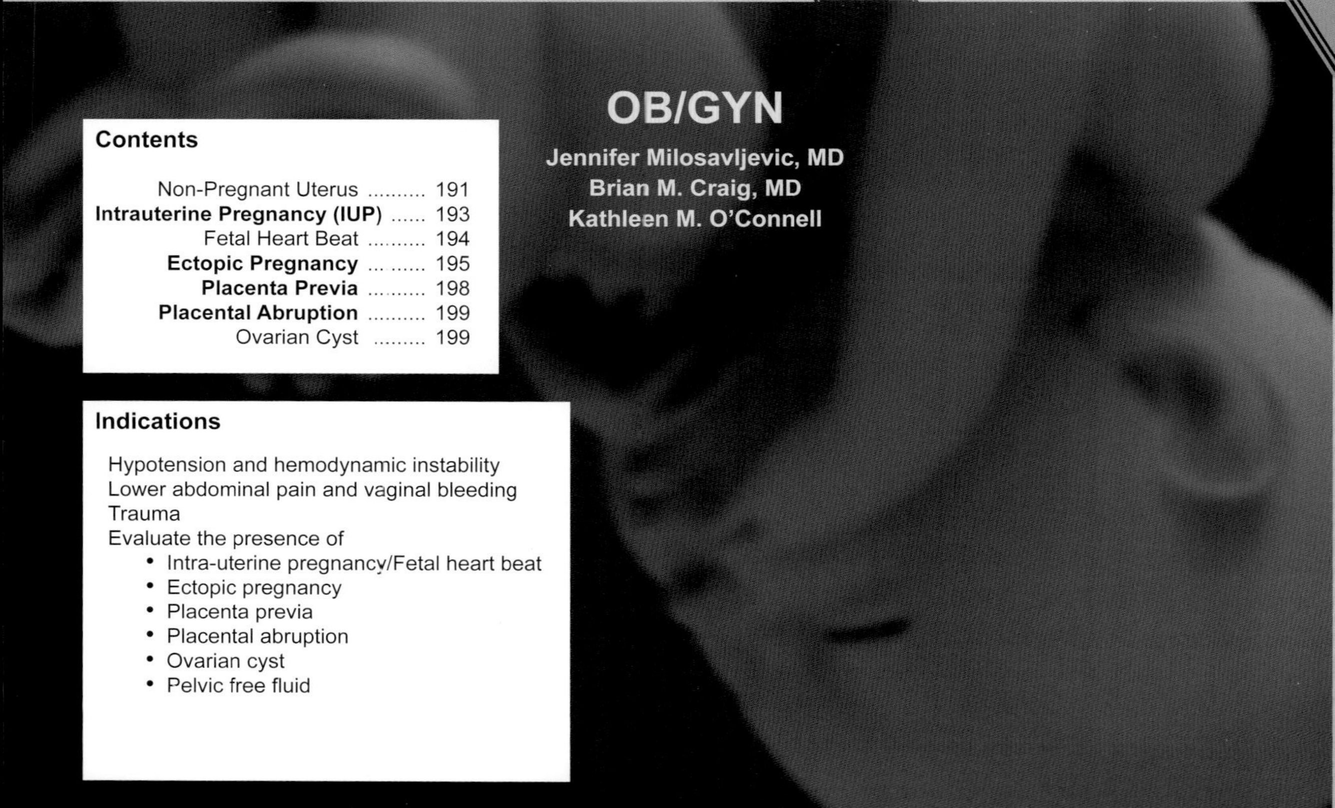

OB/GYN

Jennifer Milosavljevic, MD
Brian M. Craig, MD
Kathleen M. O'Connell

Contents

Indications

Hypotension and hemodynamic instability
Lower abdominal pain and vaginal bleeding
Trauma
Evaluate the presence of
- Intra-uterine pregnancy/Fetal heart beat
- Ectopic pregnancy
- Placenta previa
- Placental abruption
- Ovarian cyst
- Pelvic free fluid

Non-pregnant uterus

Patient position

Supine

Full bladder if possible

Transducer Type & Placement

Curvilinear 2-5 MHz

Mid line, Suprapubic, angled inferiorly

Screen marker to the left

Depth about 15-20 cm

Longitudinal/Sagittal view

- Marker cephalad
- Pan the transducer left and right to identify different structures as the uterus and ovaries

Transverse view

- Marker towards the patient's right
- Pan the transducer up and down to identify the fundus and cervix

Structures to be identified

Bladder
Uterus
Cervix & Vagina
Ovaries

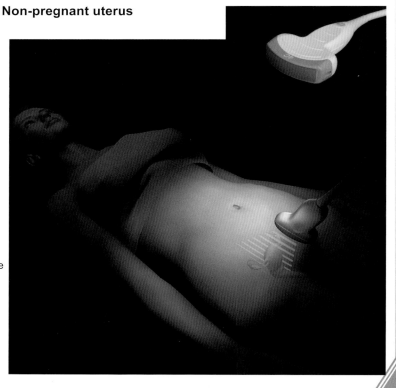

Non-pregnant uterus

Sonographic findings

Bladder

Hypoechoic structure, anterior to the uterus

Uterus

Mostly anteflexed and anteverted Located directly inferior to the bladder with grey appearance

Identify the long axis of the uterus

Normal measurements are less than 10 x 6 cm

Note the endometrial stripe and follow to the cervix

Ovaries

Can be found by panning the transducer to the right or left

Almond shaped, **slightly hypo-echoic** structures

Follicles can be seen

Normal Measurement is 2 x 2 x 3 cm

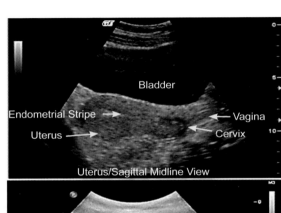

Uterus/Sagittal Midline View

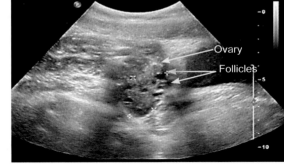

Intrauterine Pregnancy (IUP)

Structures to be identified

Gestational Sac
Fetus
Placenta
Fetal Heart beat

Gestational sac

Appears hypoechoic black inside the uterus (near the fundus) and has thickened surrounding walls

Can be visualized at 5+ weeks gestation

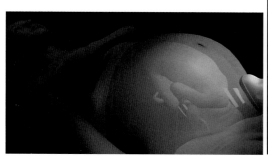

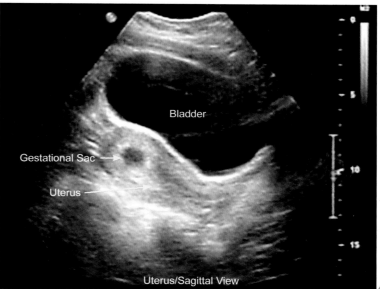

Uterus/Sagittal View

IUP/Fetal Heartbeat

Sonographic findings (cont.)

Developed **fetus** with head, body, and limbs can be seen

Placenta is usually near the fundus of the uterus and has an echo-texture similar to the liver

Confirm live IUP/Fetal Heart Beat

Can be detected from 6 weeks of gestation

Choose **M-mode** function

DO NOT USE PULSED DOPPLER. t may adversely affect the fetus

Pan the transducer to locate the heart and place the cursor over the heart beat

Measure from **peak to peak** of one or two cycles

This images demonstrates a fetal heart beat of 130bpm

A beating heart is also seen without the M-mode in the fetal thorax

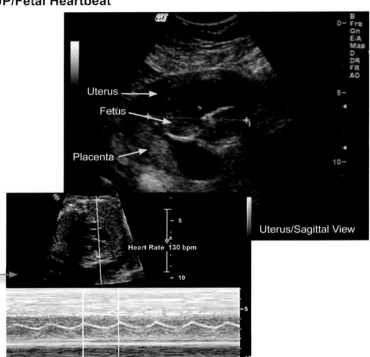

Uterus/Sagittal View

Heart Rate 130 bpm

Ectopic Pregnancy

Structures to be identified

Adnexal Mass

Ectopic gestational sac

Pseudogestational sac

Fluid in Cul-de-sac or Morrison's pouch

Sonographic findings

Finding an adnexal mass with an empty uterine cavity

Eccentric location of the gestational sac

Ectopic gestational sac and fetus with thickened wall in the fallopian tube or adnexa

The presence of **pelvic fluid** correlates with a higher possibility of ectopic pregnancy

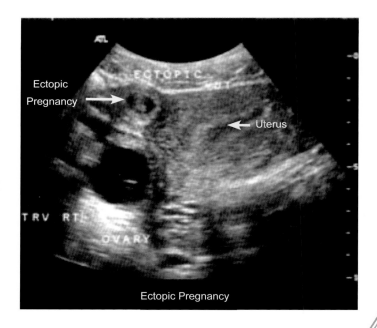

Ectopic Pregnancy

Ectopic Fluid in Morrison's Pouch

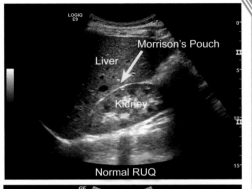

Normal RUQ

Patient position

Supine

Trendelenburg position may give a better view of the RUQ structures

Transducer Placement

About mid axillary line, 7th - 11th intercostals

Marker cephalad

Counter clock rotation help eliminate the rib shadows

Sliding the transducer downward will expose the lower edge of the liver, and the kidney, where free fluid tends to accumulate

Sliding the transducer upward will expose the right diaphragm and pleural space

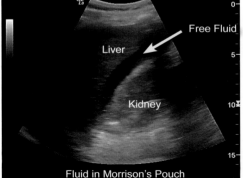

Fluid in Morrison's Pouch

Ectopic- Fluid in the Posterior Cul-de-sac

Patient Position

Supine

Transducer Placement

Suprapubic, angled inferiorly, marker cephalad
(sagittal view)

Sonographic Findings

Fluid in the cul-de-sac tend to accumulate beneath
the uterus

Gross amount usually seen with a ruptured ectopic
pregnancy

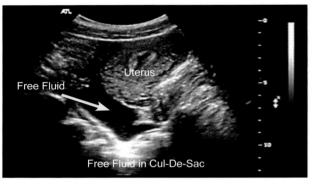

Uterus

Free Fluid

Free Fluid in Cul-De-Sac

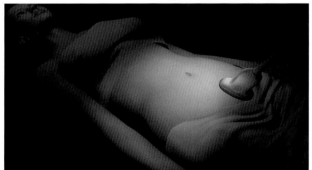

Placenta Previa

Sonographic findings

Scan is best when there are no uterine contractions

Best to start with a sagittal view to determine if the placenta is extending into the lower uterine segment

Note if the placenta is covering the **internal os**. If not, can measure the distance between the placenta and the internal os to **grade** the placenta previa

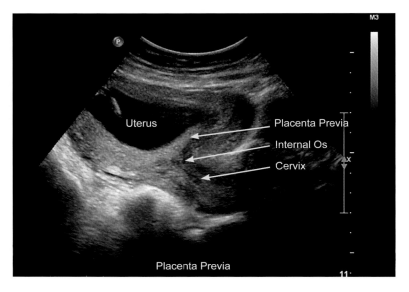

Placental Abruption

Sonographic findings

Hemorrhage within the placenta causing separation from the uterine wall

Difficult to identify with trans-abdominal ultrasound

Older hemorrhage is easier to identify

Better to start with a sagittal view

Grading is according to the location and degree of separation. Generally is termed, mild, partial and complete. Grading help determine the prognosis

Ruptured Ovarian Cyst

Sonographic findings

Locate the uterus

Pan the transducer to the sides to identify the ruptured ovarian cyst

A large **hematoma** from a ruptured ovarian cyst is sometimes visible posterior to the uterus

Not all ruptured cysts form hematomas. They could have normal shaped ovary with some **fluid collection in the cul-de-sac**

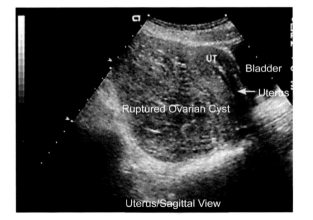

Placenta

Retro-placental Hemorrhage →

Placental Abruption

Bladder

← Uterus

UT

Ruptured Ovarian Cyst

Uterus/Sagittal View

Soft Tissue, Bone & DVT

David Amponsah, MD
Victor Coba, MD

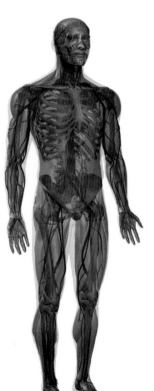

Contents

Indications

Extremity swelling, erythema, pain

Suspicion for abscess / cellulitis

Suspicion of fracture

Aid in procedures for draining abscess

Soft Tissue

Patient Position

Most critically ill patients are supine

Adjust patient position as tolerated to evaluate the affected area

Transducer type and position

Linear for superficial structures 7-13 MHz or
Curvilinear 2-5 MHz for deeper penetration

Transducer marker cephalad or towards the patient's right

Screen marker to the left of the screen

Adjust the depth according to the structure examined

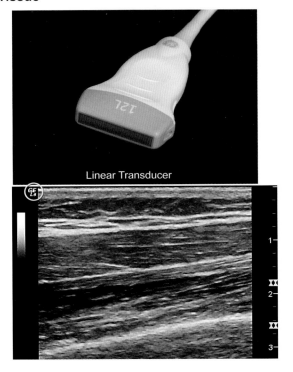

Linear Transducer

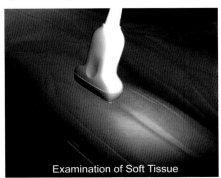

Examination of Soft Tissue

Normal Soft Tissue Structures

Exam should include sonographic evaluation of surrounding unaffected areas

Comparison to the opposite extremity

Identify:

Skin: Hyperechoic layer adjacent to the transducer

Subcutaneous tissue: hypoechoic layer of variable thickness with hyperechoic lines resembling a feather

Muscle: Feather like hypoechoic structure

Tendons: hyperechoic fibrillar structure

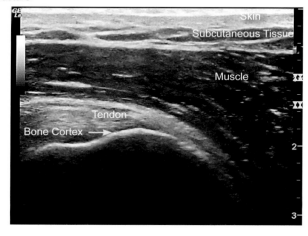

Cellulitis

Sonographic findings

Disruption of normal subcutaneous tissue echo texture resulting in **cobblestoning**

Diffuse thickening with increased echogenicity of the involved soft tissue

Edematous strands representing **distended lymphatic** channels

Findings are non specific. Skin edema or **chronic lymphedema** may have similar appearance

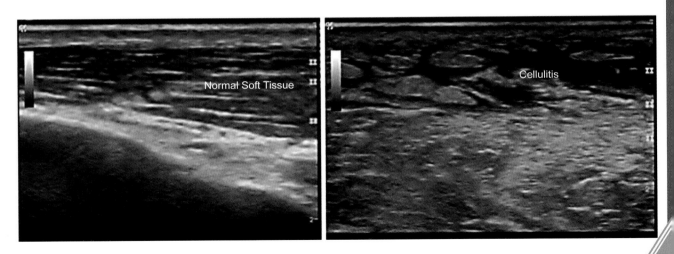

Abscess

Sonographic findings

Discrete fluid collection adjacent to a surrounding area of cellulitis

Anechoic or echogenic fluid collection with heterogeneous debris, septations or loculations

Swirling motion during ballottement (with probe compression)

Use Color Flow **(CF)** to demonstrate surrounding blood flow around periphery

Rule out vascular structures with color or PW Doppler

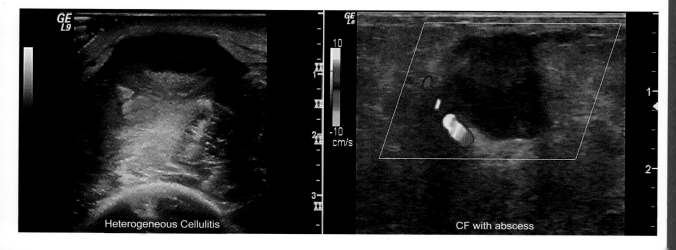

Heterogeneous Cellulitis   CF with abscess

Bones

Patient position

Supine

Place transducer at the location of pain

Transducer Type & Placement

Linear 7-13 MHz

Transducer marker pointing cephalad or
towards the patient's right

Screen marker located to the left of the screen

Depth 5-10 cm depending on the structure examined
or the patient's body habitus

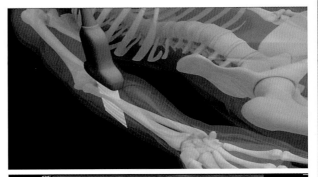

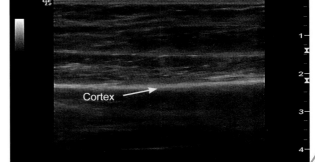

Cortex

Fractures

Sonographic findings

Obtain short and long axis of the bony cortex

Identify the bony acoustic surface **(cortex)**

Evaluate for any cortical irregularities or interruptions

Evaluate for any hypoechoic hematoma adjacent to the fracture site

Evaluate the opposite extremity if possible for normal variants as comparison.

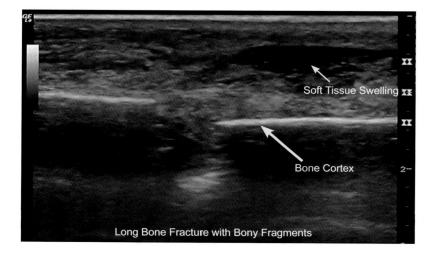

Long Bone Fracture with Bony Fragments

Patient Position

Femoral Veins

- Supine, hip in slight flexion and external rotation

Popliteal Vein

- Supine, leg flexed at the knee with external rotation

Transducer Type & Placement

Linear 7-13 MHz

Transducer marker towards the patient's right

Screen marker on the left side of the screen

Depth 5-10 cm depending on the patient's size

Three Point Compression Technique includes evaluation of areas of the highest turbulence and greatest risk for developing a thrombus

- **Common femoral vein (CFV)** at the saphenofemoral junction
- **Proximal deep Femoral Vein (DFV)** and the superficial femoral vein (SFV)
- **Popliteal Vein**

Non-visualization of a clot does not rule out a DVT (False negative - may not be echogenic depending on the gain adjustment or auto gain)

Do not confuse a **Baker's cyst** with a blood vessel (evaluate with color Doppler)

DVT

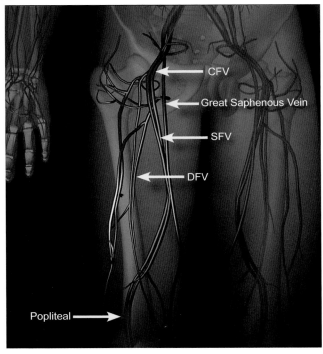

DVT

Sonographic Findings

Common Femoral Vein (CFV)

Start at the inguinal ligament and scan to the superior calf 2 cm at a time

First find the junction of the **saphenous vein** and **CFV**

Differentiate between the artery and the vein, using Color Flow **(CF)** and Pulse Wave **(PW)** Doppler if necessary

Apply gentle compression initially, so as not to collapse the vein completely (enough pressure is when the artery **starts** to deform)

Obtain long and short axis views

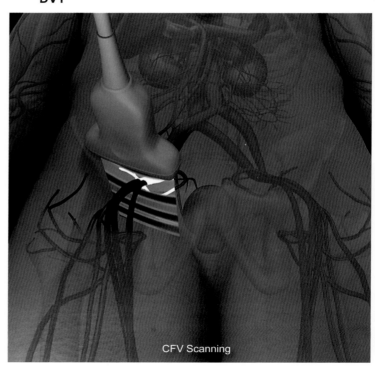

CFV Scanning

DVT

Sonographic Findings (cont.)
CFV

Gray scale compression is considered the most useful in the diagnosis of DVT

- Compression of the vein to the point of collapse

- Involves compression of the calf muscles distal to the vein examined. This will create **venous augmentation** noted on the gray scale image

- Apply the PW Doppler and color Doppler to note the augmentation as a pulse wave or blush of color respectively

- Note the **Phasic variation**: variation in venous flow with respiration. This can be noted by applying PW Doppler

- Venous augmentation mostly indicate the vein patency between the level of the compression and the US transducer

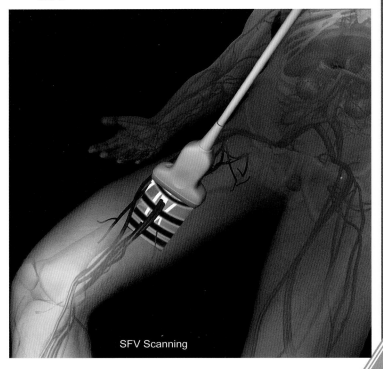

SFV Scanning

DVT

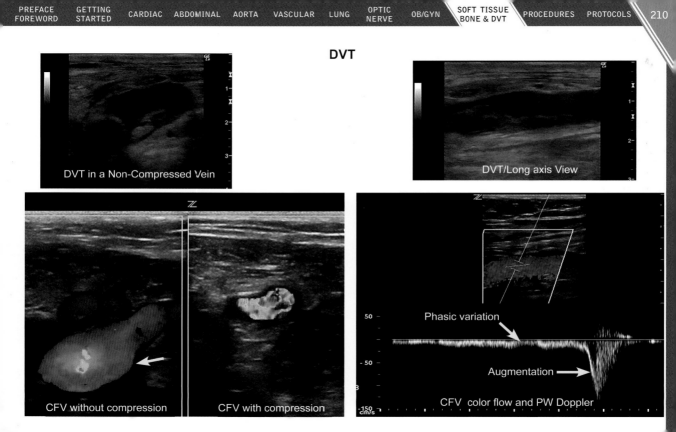

DVT in a Non-Compressed Vein

DVT/Long axis View

CFV without compression

CFV with compression

Phasic variation

Augmentation

CFV color flow and PW Doppler

DVT

Sonographic Findings (cont.)
DFV & SFV

- Identify and scan the DFV and the SFV (the SFV is a deep vein, also known as the femoral vein)

- Chronic DVT(s) tend to adhere to the vessel wall

- Continue scanning the mid and distal femoral veins

- If a DVT is found, it is advisable to measure its extent. Long axis view can help

- Store a still image of the DVT

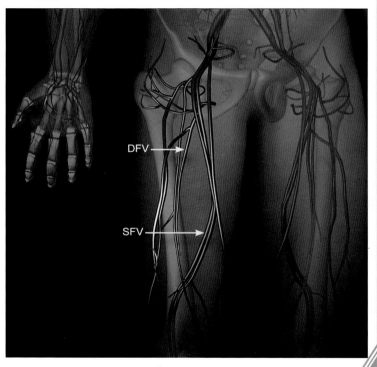

DVT

Sonographic Findings

Popliteal Vein

- Place transducer in the transverse orientation in the popliteal fossa and identify the popliteal vein which is superficial to the popliteal artery

- Perform Gray Scale Compression with augmentation by pressure on the calf and apply color Doppler and PW Doppler during augmentation

- Differentiate from a Baker's cyst by applying CF

- Note the phasic variation and augmentation

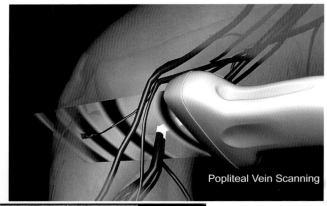

Popliteal Vein Scanning

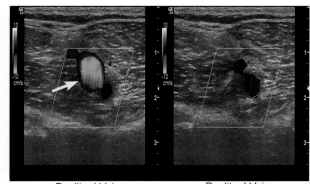

Popliteal Vein without compression

Popliteal Vein with compression

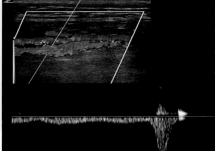

Long Axis/Popliteal Vein with color flow and PW Doppler showing phasic variation and positive augmentation

Worksheet

Patient Name: _____

MRN: _____

Date: _____

History: _____

Common Femoral vein and Proximal Greater Saphenous Vein

Compressible   ☐ Y   ☐ N

Color Flow   ☐ Y   ☐ N

Augmentation   ☐ Y   ☐ N

Proximal Deep Femoral Vein and Superficial Femoral Vein

Compressible   ☐ Y   ☐ N

Color Flow   ☐ Y   ☐ N

Augmentation   ☐ Y   ☐ N

Mid Femoral Vein

Compressible   ☐ Y   ☐ N

Color Flow   ☐ Y   ☐ N

Augmentation   ☐ Y   ☐ N

Popliteal Vein

Compressible   ☐ Y   ☐ N

Color Flow   ☐ Y   ☐ N

Augmentation   ☐ Y   ☐ N

Impression & Comments:

Procedures

Victor Coba, MD
Keith Killu, MD

Contents

Transducer Types

Choose the transducer according to the structure depth and location. For **deeper structures** a lower frequency transducer is used. Higher frequency transducers provide better axial resolution

Procedures/Patient Position & Prescan

Position the patient in the standard optimal position, (e.g. Internal Jugular Vein access, place the patient in Trendelenburg position) If using ultrasound to mark a location only, make sure the patient stays in the same position

The ultrasound machine is placed where the operator can **easily visualize** the screen

Perform a prescan of the structure prior to the sterilization process

Choose a site where the structure is larger and closer to the skin if possible

Adjust the **depth and gain**

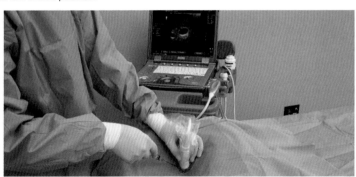

Sterility

Sterile kit usually includes

- **Sterile sheath and gel**
- **Rubber bands**
- **Needle guides** with different angle paths for different depths

Place **gel** inside the sterile sheath

Place the **sterile sheath** on the transducer head and roll the sheath along the entire transducer cable

Place the **rubber bands**, one near the head and the other near the base of the transducer

Place sterile gel outside the sheath along the transducer head

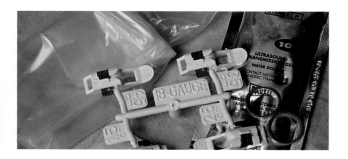

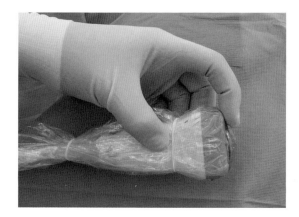

Needle Guide

Use a **Needle Guide** if desired

Included in most sterile kits
The needle guide is to be attached to the transducer head
The needle tip is introduced through the guide

Advantages:

- Predictable path, depth and angle of the needle
- Less hand eye coordination is needed

Disadvantages:

- The angle is fixed
- Deeper structures are hard to reach

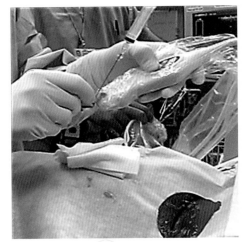

Orientation

The **screen marker is placed to the left** of the screen. **The transducer marker is placed to the right of the patient.**
Make sure the marker side corresponds to the left side of the screen by touching the transducer footprint near the transducer marker

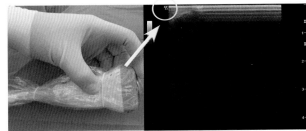

Procedure

General Procedure Steps

Locate the structure to be accessed and apply local anaesthesia

Place the needle behind the transducer at about **1-2 cm**

Perform an **imitation poke** and notice the **ring down** artifact, acoustic shadowing to locate the needle

Needle angle is usually about **45°-60°** from the skin. Can change the angle when trying to avoid another structure

Insertion method

Move the needle in slow short controlled strokes and monitor it's progress

Locate the **tip** of the needle (which may appear as an echogenic dot)

Place the **bevel** towards the transducer beam, where this can produce more echo return and better visualization of the needle tip

Be sure not to mistake the shaft for the tip of the needle

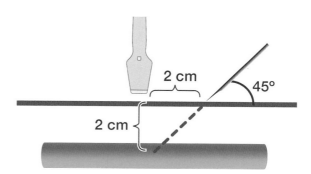

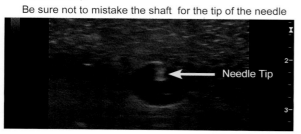

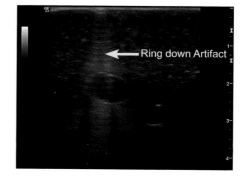

Thoracentesis

Patient Position
Most ICU patients will be in a supine position

Arm abducted and flexed at the elbow

Consider elevating the head of the bed

Transducer type & Placement
Phased Array 2.5-5 MHz

Transducer marker pointing cephalad

Depth about 15 cm

Transducer Placement and Views
L3/Place the transducer in the mid or posterior axillary line near the RUQ or LUQ to identify the **diaphragm**

Scan the whole area from the anterior chest to the posterior axillary line

Scan at least 3 intercostal spaces

If the patient can sit, they should face away from the operator and the scan should include the area from the scapula down to the posterior thoracic ribs, and from the paravertebral to the posterior axillary lines **(L4)**. Try to locate the largest area of effusion

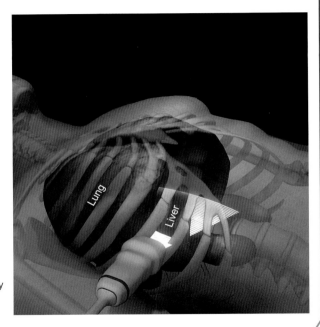

Thoracentesis

Transducer Placement and Views (cont.)

Locate the diaphragm, liver, or spleen which are excellent land marks for ultrasound

Procedure

Note the depth of the fluid

A 15 mm fluid thickness between the visceral and parietal pleura over three intercostal spaces is usually enough to try a thoracentesis

Mid or posterior axillary line is usually optimal

Supply adequate anesthesia

Complete sterility

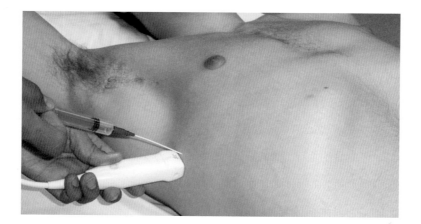

Thoracentesis

Procedure (cont.)

Place the needle beside the transducer and follow its path with real time guidance

Real time US guidance is not always necessary

Keep the patient in the same position after the prescan

Perform the procedure following the standard techniques

Catheter tip can be identified inside the pleural fluid

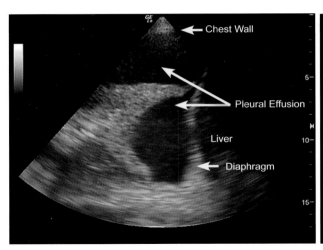

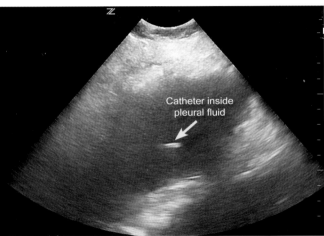

Paracentesis

Patient Position

Patient in a supine or left lateral oblique position if choosing the LLQ

Consider raising the head of the bed if possible

Transducer type & Placement

Curvilinear 2-5MHz

Transducer marker towards the patient's right

Procedure

Prescan the lower part of the abdomen, identifying the largest fluid accumulation

LLQ not necessarily the best, but usually the better position

Avoid upper quadrants and rectus muscle

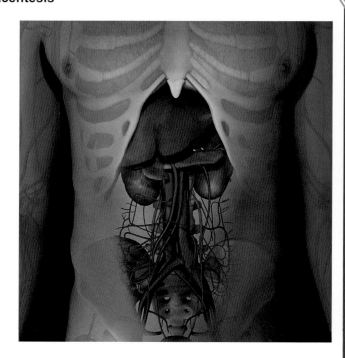

Paracentesis

Procedure (cont.)

Identify the **free floating bowel** and the bladder to avoid injury

A collection of at least 3-4 cm in depth (distance between the abdominal wall and the floating bowel loops) is usually adequate for paracentesis

Scan the fluid collection in long and short axis

Ascitic fluid could have varying degrees of echogenicity characteristics. Bladder fluid is usually anechoeic

Locate the largest pocket of fluid to perform the procedure

Avoid when adhesions are present

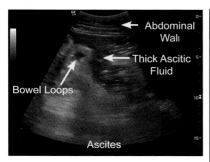

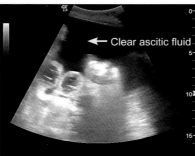

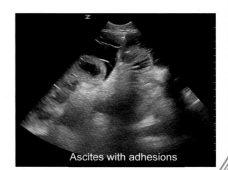

Paracentesis

Procedure (cont.)

Needle angle should be 60-90° to the skin, placed close and behind the transducer

Success rates is about 95%

Perform the rest of the procedure following the standard technique and sterility with the aid of US guidance and sterile sheath kit

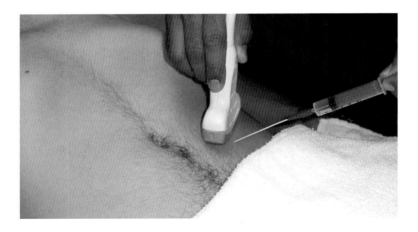

Suprapubic Bladder Aspiration

Patient Position

Supine

Head of bed better at 30° if possible

Transducer type & Placement

Curvilinear 2-5 MHz

A7/ Place the transducer directly above the pubic symphysis pointing inferiorly towards the pelvis

> ### Long axis
> Transducer marker cephalad
>
> ### Short axis
> Transducer marker towards the patient's right

Views and Procedure

Bladder fluid is usually **anechoic**

Differentiate the bladder from

- Any **distended bowel**, which usually have **peristalsis**
- Identify any large ovarian cysts
- Ureteral jets can help differentiate structures by using Color Flow

Success rate increase when transverse diameter is > 3.5 cm

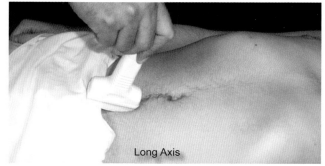

Long Axis

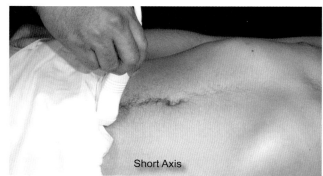

Short Axis

Suprapubic Bladder Aspiration

Procedure (cont.)

Place the needle beside the transducer and follow its path with real time guidance

Real time US guidance is not always necessary

Keep the patient in the same position after the prescan

Perform the procedure following the standard techniques

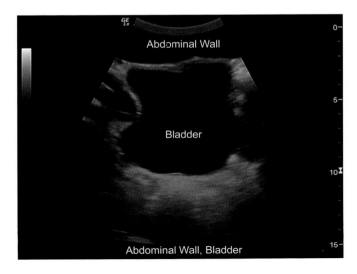

Lumbar Puncture

Patient Position

Patient in the lateral decubitus position with the knees and back flexed

If possible a sitting position with the patient leaning forward

Transducer type & Placement

Curvilinear 2-5MHz or linear

Transducer placed over the spinous processes of choosing, **L2-L5**

Depth about 8 cm

Sagittal Axis

- Transducer marker cephalad

Short Axis

- Transducer marker towards the patient's right

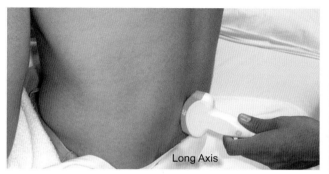

Long Axis

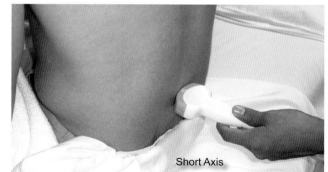

Short Axis

Lumbar Puncture

Views and Procedure

Spinous processes above and below the desired space should be identified

Start with a transverse view to identify the midline, then obtain a longitudinal view

The spinous process appears as a hyperechoic round edge structure

Transducer moved superiorly and inferiorly between the spinous processes to identify the interspinous spaces and the path for needle advancement

Between the spaces, the ligamentum flavum (with hyper-echoic thin lines) is followed by the Dura matter

Real time ultrasound guidance is not always needed or preferred. Apply local anasthesia

Perform the rest of the procedure in the standard sterile technique

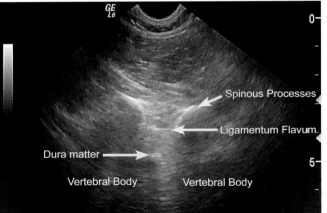

Spinous Processes

Ligamentum Flavum

Dura matter

Vertebral Body   Vertebral Body

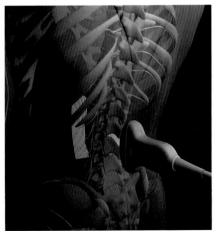

Pericardiocentesis

Patient Position

Patient in a supine position

Transducer Type & Placement

Curvilinear or phased array transducer

A1/ Subxiphoid is the better view

Left parasternal long axis is best for detecting posterior effusions

Depth about 15 cm

Views and Procedure

The subxiphoid is commonly used to perform the procedure

- Transducer just inferior to the xiphoid process and pointing towards the left costal margin

Choose the site where the effusion is maximal and is closest to the skin

Note the depth of the effusion

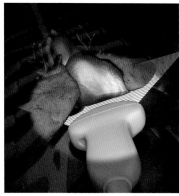

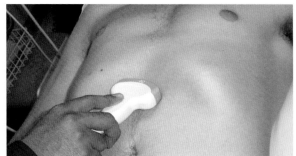

Pericardiocentesis

Views and Procedure (cont.)

Make sure the track of the needle is clear. i.e. avoiding the **lung and liver**

Attention to avoid the **internal mammary** (3-5 mm on the left of sternal border) and the neurovascular bundle at the inferior edge of the ribs

Use US prior to insertion but not for actual guidance during the procedure

Note the trajectory of the ultrasound beam, which represents the trajectory of the needle

Apply local anesthesia

18 gauge angiocath is usually used

Procedure to be done following the standard guidelines

Can confirm the angiocath presence in the pericardial sac by ultrasound

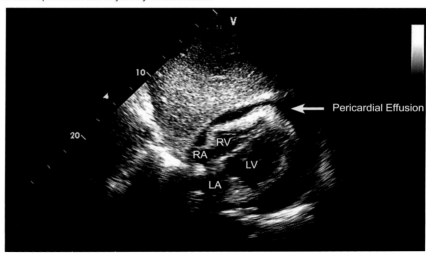

Tracheostomy & Endotracheal (ET) Intubation

Patient Position
Supine

Transducer type & Placement
Linear 7-13 MHz

Short Axis
- Marker towards the patient's right

Long Axis
- Marker cephalad

Structures to be identified
Thyroid and cricoid cartilage

Thyroid gland (Isthmus)

Tracheal rings

Blood Vessels

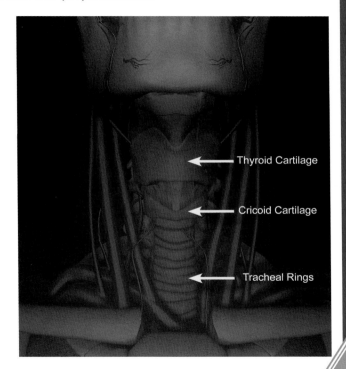

Thyroid Cartilage

Cricoid Cartilage

Tracheal Rings

Tracheostomy & Endotracheal (ET) Intubation

Procedure and Views
Tracheostomy

Procedure to be performed following the standard technique

Pre procedure ultrasound will help

- Identify tracheal and paratracheal tissue and blood vessels
- Identify the depth of the trachea
- Choose best incision site

US can be used during the procedure for guidance

ET intubation

US can be used post intubation to confirm the ET tube inside the trachea

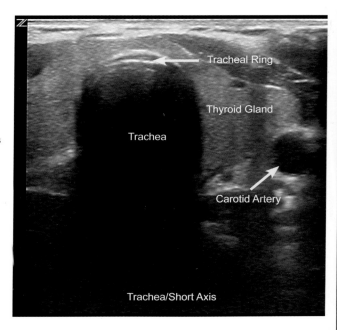

Tracheostomy & Endotracheal (ET) Intubation

Procedure and Views (cont.)

Inflated cuff

- Find the cuff by angling the transducer inferiorly
- Appears more echogenic
- Acoustic shadowing can be seen
- Inflating and deflating the balloon will create a sliding motion

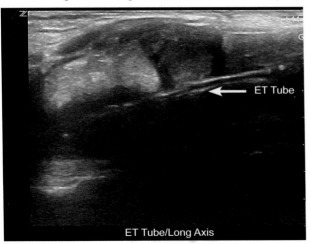

ET Tube/Long Axis

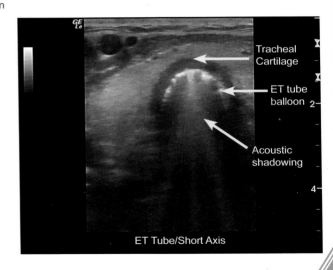

Tracheal Cartilage

ET tube balloon

Acoustic shadowing

ET Tube/Short Axis

Clinical Protocols

Luca Neri, MD
Enrico Storti, MD
Gabriele Via, MD
Thanks to Daniel Lichtenstein
for his guidance and inspiration

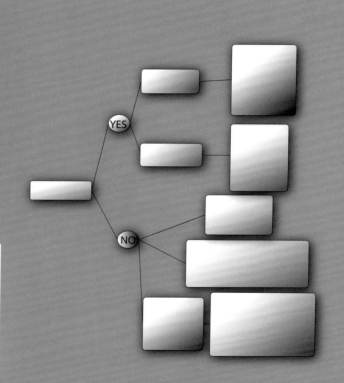

Contents

Table 1 - Ultrasound Life Support WINFOCUS Pathways

ABCDE: Multi-focused Ultrasound

	A Airway	B Breathing	C Circulation	D Disability	E Expose, Exclude Extend to Head-to-toes
1	**Cervical US** Subcutaneous emphysema hematomas	**Lung US** Atelectasis Pulmonary edema Pneumonia, Contusion	**Echo** Cardiac function Pericardial fluid Pulmonary embolism Procedures	**Ocular US** ONSD, Pupillary reflexes, Emphysema, Retinal Detachment	**Head & Other** Ocular, skull, cervical, pelvis, limbs Procedures & Monitor
2	Trachea patency, placement & lesions ET Device patency & placement	**Pleural US** Sq. emphysema Pneumothorax Pleural fluid Procedures	**Vascular US** IVC , AAA, DVT, Access **MSK US** Hematomas, Fractures	**Cranial US** Trans-cranial Doppler Midline shift Fractures	**Thorax US** Advanced ECHO, lung, mediastinum, Procedures & Monitor
3	**Lung US** Subcutaneous emphysema Dynamic lung artifacts	**Echo/Vascular US** Cardiac function, DVT **Diaphragm US** Paralysis, Injuries	**Abdominal US** FAST, Hematomas **OB/GYN US** Ectopic, Hematomas	**Diaphragm US** Paralysis/Paresis [Cervical lesion]	**Abdominal US** Visceral & parenchymal organs, Retro-peritoneum, Procedures

Table A - Airway Focused Ultrasound

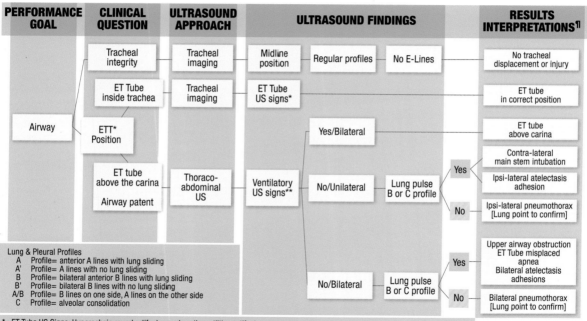

Lung & Pleural Profiles
- A   Profile= anterior A lines with lung sliding
- A'   Profile= A lines with no lung sliding
- B   Profile= bilateral anterior B lines with lung sliding
- B'   Profile= bilateral B lines with no lung sliding
- A/B   Profile= B lines on one side, A lines on the other side
- C   Profile= alveolar consolidation

* ET Tube US Signs: Hyperechoic round artifact, reverberations, tilting artifacts
** Thoraco-abdominal Ventilatory US Signs: Lung sliding, Dynamic air bronchogram, B/C lines or Consolidation movements, Fluid movements
¶ Likely diagnosis. Prefer and continue with the corresponding protocol. Always confirm results clinically.

Table B Breathing Focused Ultrasound

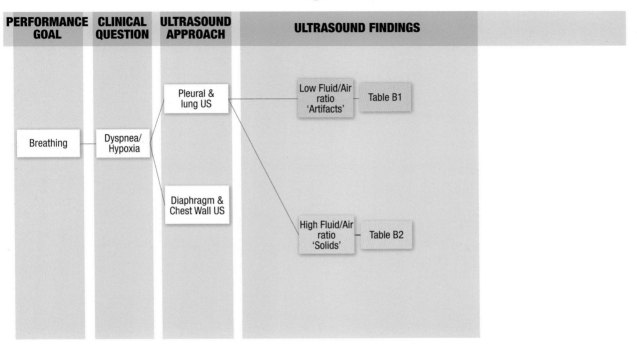

PERFORMANCE GOAL	CLINICAL QUESTION	ULTRASOUND APPROACH	ULTRASOUND FINDINGS	

Breathing

Dyspnea/ Hypoxia

Pleural & lung US

Diaphragm & Chest Wall US

Low Fluid/Air ratio 'Artifacts' — Table B1

High Fluid/Air ratio 'Solids' — Table B2

Table B.1 - Breathing Focused Ultrasound

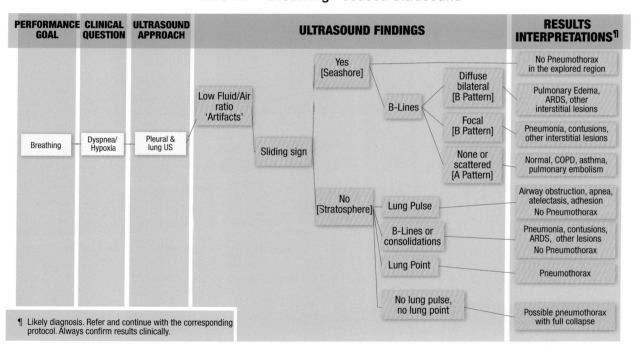

¶ Likely diagnosis. Refer and continue with the corresponding protocol. Always confirm results clinically.

Table B.2 - Breathing Focused Ultrasound

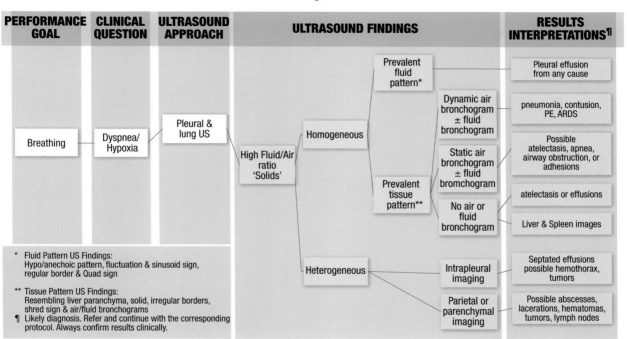

PERFORMANCE GOAL	CLINICAL QUESTION	ULTRASOUND APPROACH	ULTRASOUND FINDINGS			RESULTS INTERPRETATIONS¶
Breathing	Dyspnea/ Hypoxia	Pleural & lung US	High Fluid/Air ratio 'Solids'	Homogeneous	Prevalent fluid pattern*	Pleural effusion from any cause
					Dynamic air bronchogram ± fluid bronchogram	pneumonia, contusion, PE, ARDS
					Static air bronchogram ± fluid bromchogram	Possible atelectasis, apnea, airway obstruction, or adhesions
				Prevalent tissue pattern**	No air or fluid bronchogram	atelectasis or effusions
						Liver & Spleen images
				Heterogeneous	Intrapleural imaging	Septated effusions possible hemothorax, tumors
					Parietal or parenchymal imaging	Possible abscesses, lacerations, hematomas, tumors, lymph nodes

* Fluid Pattern US Findings:
Hypo/anechoic pattern, fluctuation & sinusoid sign, regular border & Quad sign

** Tissue Pattern US Findings:
Resembling liver paranchyma, solid, irregular borders, shred sign & air/fluid bronchograms

¶ Likely diagnosis. Refer and continue with the corresponding protocol. Always confirm results clinically.

Table B.3 Dyspnea Multi-focused Ultrasound

Dyspnea Patterns	Pneumonia	Pulmonary Embolism	Pneumothorax	Pulmonary Edema	Lung Contusion
Heart	± Pericardial Fluid	RV dilated, hypokinetic, paradoxical IVS	RV small, hyperkinetic	+/- LV dilated, LV hypokinetic ± valvular dysfunction	Variable
IVC	Variable	Fixed & distended	Fixed & distended	Fixed & distended	Variable
Lung	Focal B or B', ±Shred sign, ± dynamic air bronchogram, ± pleural effusion	A Profile Lung pulse, ± Consolidation	A' Profile ± Lung Point ±E Lines	B Profile Lung pulse, ± Pleural Fluid	Focal B or B', Shred sign, ± dynamic air bronchogram, ± pleural fluid
Others	± Reduced diaphragm movement	±Vein thrombosis, Distended hepatic veins	±Tracheal displacement, distended hepatic veins	±Distended hepatic veins	±Pleural or peritoneal fluid

Table B.3 Dyspnea Multi-focused Ultrasound (cont.)

Dyspnea Patterns	COPD	Asthma	Chronic Interstitial Disease	ARDS	Upper Airway Obstruction Atelectasis ETT Displacement
Heart	Variable RV dilated & hypertrophic	Variable	Variable RV dilated & hypertrophic	Variable RV dilated & hypokinetic	Variable
IVC	Variable	Variable	Variable	Variable	Variable
Lung	A Profile lung pulse, ± ↓ Sliding	A Profile lung pulse, ± ↓ Sliding	B Profile lung pulse ± ↓ Sliding	B/C Profile, lung pulse, ± ↓ Sliding, ± dynamic air bronchogram ± fluid	Bi/Uni-lateral A Profile, lung pulse, ± ↓↓↓ Sliding, ± static air bronchogram
Others	---	---	---	---	↓Diaphragm movement ± esophageal ETT placement

Table C Shock Focused Echocardiography

Shock State

Pre Existing Cardiac Disease	Focused Echo Findings		Potential Clinical Diagnosis
I	LV and LA dilatation	Yes	Dilated Cardiomyopathy
II	LV hypertrophy	Yes	Hypertrophic Obstructive Cardiomyopathy, Aortic Stenosis, Hypertensive Cardiomyopathy…
III	RV dilatation ± hypertrophy	Yes	Chronic Cor Pulmonale

IVC

< 1 cm & Inspiratory collapse >50% during spontaneous breathing < 1-1.5 cm & Inspiratory distention >20% during passive mechanical ventilation	Hypovolemia	Confirm diagnosis with small hyperkinetic RV & LV
1.5-2.5 cm with respiratory variation Inspiratory collapse <50% with spontaneous breathing	Normal/Inconclusive, Consider Vasoplesia or Hypovolemia if I, II,or III positive	
Dilated and fixed IVC	Possible RV failure, Tamponade, Fluid overload	

Table C Shock Focused Echocardiography (cont.)

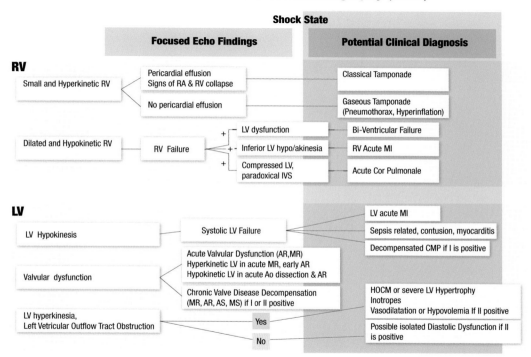

Shock State

Focused Echo Findings | **Potential Clinical Diagnosis**

RV

Small and Hyperkinetic RV
- Pericardial effusion / Signs of RA & RV collapse → Classical Tamponade
- No pericardial effusion → Gaseous Tamponade (Pneumothorax, Hyperinflation)

Dilated and Hypokinetic RV → RV Failure
- + LV dysfunction → Bi-Ventricular Failure
- +/- Inferior LV hypo/akinesia → RV Acute MI
- + Compressed LV, paradoxical IVS → Acute Cor Pulmonale

LV

LV Hypokinesis → Systolic LV Failure
- LV acute MI
- Sepsis related, contusion, myocarditis
- Decompensated CMP if I is positive

Valvular dysfunction
- Acute Valvular Dysfunction (AR,MR) / Hyperkinetic LV in acute MR, early AR / Hypokinetic LV in acute Ao dissection & AR
- Chronic Valve Disease Decompensation (MR, AR, AS, MS) if I or II positive

LV hyperkinesia, Left Vetricular Outflow Tract Obstruction
- Yes → HOCM or severe LV Hypertrophy / Inotropes / Vasodilatation or Hypovolemia If II positive
- No → Possible isolated Diastolic Dysfunction if II is positive

Table C1 Shock Multi-focused Ultrasound

Shock & PEA Patterns	Cardiac Tamponade	Pulmonary Embolism	Tension Pneumothorax	Heart Failure	Hypovolemia ± Low Peripheral Resistance
Heart	RV small & hyperkinetic, pericardial effusion	RV dilated & hypokinetic, systolic paradoxical IVS	RV small & hyperkinetic	+/- LV dilated, LV hypokinetic ± valvular dysfunction	LV & RV small & hyperkinetic
IVC	Fixed & distended	Fixed & distended	Fixed & distended	Fixed & distended	Flexible & Collapsing
Lung	A Profile	A Profile ± Consolidation	A' Profile ± Lung Point	B Profile ± Pleural Fluid	A Profile
Others	Distended hepatic veins	Vein thrombosis, distended hepatic veins	± Tracheal displacement, distended hepatic veins	Distended hepatic veins	± Peritoneal or retroperitoneal fluid, ± AAA ± Septic Foci

Suggested Readings

General Ultrasound and the Critically Ill, D. Lichtenstein

The Echo Manual, Jae K. Oh

Emergency Ultrasound, O. John Ma

Ultrasound Scanning, Principals and Protocols, Betty Tempktin

Diagnostic and Surgical Imaging Anatomy, Ahuja

Critical Care Ultrasonography, A. Levitov

http://www.winfocus.org/abcde

This handbook of CU ultrasound is an excellent example of the Earth based benefits of space medical research. The National Space Biomedical Research Institute supports research to develop intuitive educational programs to train astronauts to perform ultrasound examinations on the International Space Station; this handbook is a direct extension of that successful research project and provides a very useful guide to ultrasound use in the Intensive Care Unit.

Jeffrey Sutton, MD, PhD • Director • National Space Biomedical Research Institute

Real-time ultrasound at the point-of-care, has become an invaluable adjunct to the clinical management of critically ill and injured patients both for pre- and in-hospital settings. The rate at which it is spreading, and the continuing development of new applications, may outpace training of adequate numbers of qualified users.

WINFOCUS, the World Interactive Network Focused on Critical UltraSound, is fully committed to enhance and spread quality in the field, through appropriate Education, Clinical Research, Technology Development, Networking, and is eager to support editorial initiatives like this one.

This new handy pocket-book is the ideal reference to consult when making bedside or on-scene interpretations of ultrasound clinical data, mostly when integrated either into time-dependent, crowdy, remote or scarce-resource scenarios. Developed according to a multiple goal–oriented, patient-centred, easy-to-use style, it fully addresses the approach of critical and intensive care professionals, who typically deal with acute, unstable or complex states, rather than individual organ complaints.

This manual is another great tool to make ultrasound accessible worldwide, at the point-of-care of any emergency or critical patient.

Luca Neri, MD • USCME Project Director, WINFOCUS • Past President, WINFOCUS

ISBN: 978-0-615-35560-3 **89.95 US**

5 8 9 9 5

9 780615 355603